URBAN HEALTH SERVICES

URBAN HEALTH SERVICES

THE CASE OF NEW YORK

by ELI GINZBERG
AND THE CONSERVATION OF
HUMAN RESOURCES STAFF
COLUMBIA UNIVERSITY

COLUMBIA UNIVERSITY PRESS
NEW YORK AND LONDON   1971

For

My physician friends—practitioners,
teachers, and researchers

who helped me to gain perspective about
things medical

In appreciation and gratitude

PREFACE

THE PRESENT STUDY is the most recent in a continuing research effort that the Conservation of Human Resources Project of Columbia University has been carrying on for the New York City Planning Commission. Earlier publications include:

> *Electronic Data Processing in New York City: Lessons for Metropolitan Economics,* by Boris Yavitz and Thomas M. Stanback, 1967

> *Manpower Strategy for the Metropolis,* by Eli Ginzberg and the Conservation of Human Resources Staff, Columbia University, 1968

The selection of urban health services as the focus of the present inquiry can readily be explained. With New York City spending about $1 billion annually on health services; with clear and unequivocal evidence that much is awry with its municipal hospital system; with unsettlement introduced as a result of Medicare and Medicaid; with insistence from the community that it play a larger role in decisions affecting health planning; with the health services industry representing one of the fastest growing arenas of employment, particularly for members of minority groups—for these as well as other reasons—the interest of the Planning Commission in a critical assessment of the decision-making mechanism in the health field is obvious.

Less obvious is the fact that the subject represents a confluence of several of the Conservation staff's long-term interests. Medical economics has long been an area of our concern, as witnessed by earlier publications of the project:

A Program for the Nursing Profession (1948)
A Pattern for Hospital Care (1949)
Planning for Better Hospital Care (1961)
Allied Health Manpower (1969)
Men, Money, and Medicine (1969)

Moreover, since the publication of *The Pluralistic Economy* in 1964 the Conservation staff has continued to explore the ways in which the private, nonprofit, and governmental sectors are inter-related in the production and distribution of critical goods and services. Medical care is an outstanding illustration of this new pluralism.

Both as theoreticians and as citizens, members of the Conservation staff were intrigued with the reasons for the very slow implementation of many well-supported recommendations for far-reaching changes in the health system. The subject of *Effecting Change in Large Organizations* had attracted the staff's attention earlier (1957) and a new inquiry into the decision-making process in the urban health system offered a further opportunity for the staff to study this critical arena.

We have noted in the chapters which follow the principal sources on which we drew for information and enlightenment. A selective bibliography has been prepared.

In addition we want to acknowledge the special assistance we received from the staffs of the following organizations:

The New York City Planning Commission
Health and Hospital Planning Council of Southern New York, Inc.
United Hospital Fund of New York
Bureau of Records and Statistics, Department of Health, Health Services Administration
Medical Statistics Office, Department of Hospitals, Health Services Administration
Office of Medical Economics, Department of Health of the State of New York
Office of the Chancellor, City University of New York

The following individuals were particularly helpful:

Dr. Howard Brown, Misericordia Hospital, Bronx

Mrs. Marilyn Einhorn, Health Insurance Plan of Greater New York

Dean William Glazier, Albert Einstein College of Medicine of Yeshiva University

Dr. Marcus Kogel, Yeshiva University

Mr. Herbert Lukashok, Albert Einstein College of Medicine of Yeshiva University

Mrs. Joan Leiman, Bureau of the Budget, New York City

Assistant Commissioner Henry Manning, Department of Hospitals

Dr. Beatrice Mintz, School of Public Health and Administrative Medicine, Columbia University

Professor Charlotte Muller, Center for Social Research, City University of New York

Mrs. Nora Piore, Association for the Aid of Crippled Children

Assistant Commissioner Henry Rosner, Department of Social Services

Dr. Paul Torrens, St. Luke's Hospital Center

Dr. Ray E. Trussell, Beth Israel Medical Center

Mrs. Dorothy Woodhead, Health and Hospital Planning Council of Southern New York, Inc.

Mr. Paul Worthington, Center for Social Research, City University of New York

As the contents page indicates, Mrs. Miriam Ostow and Mr. Charles Brecher were the most actively involved of the Conservation staff in the present undertaking. Mrs. Ostow served as my principal collaborator. Her insightful and critical judgment turned many tentative leads into solid accomplishments.

We are grateful to Professor Herbert E. Klarman of New York University for making time in his busy schedule to read and criticize the manuscript, as a result of which we were able to correct and improve it.

Mrs. Ruth Szold Ginzberg edited the manuscript and read the proof and in the process made the book more readable.

ELI GINZBERG, *Director*
Conservation of Human Resources Project

CONTENTS

TABLES

FIGURES

CHARTS

CONTENTS

MAPS

URBAN HEALTH SERVICES

INTRODUCTION:
THE CHANGING MEDICAL
SCENE

THIS INTRODUCTORY CHAPTER will suggest why our investigation of the health services in New York City was undertaken and will present the range of problems on which the research was focused. The two concluding chapters will set out the lessons that can be extracted. First, however, we will define the parameters of the changes that have been occurring in New York City during the past two decades with particular attention to critical developments in the provision of medical services.

To begin with, the flow of people into and out of the city. During these years, earlier trends continued: many white middle-class families moved to the suburbs and their places were taken by a rapidly growing Negro and Puerto Rican population, the combined result of natural increase and in-migration. From 1950 to the end of the 1960s this shifting resulted in an estimated net decline of 1.3 million whites and a net increase of an equal number of Negroes and Puerto Ricans. In 1970, whites constituted 70 percent, Negroes and Puerto Ricans 30 percent, of the city's population, which has remained almost a constant 7.8 million throughout the last two decades.

The following consequences can be traced directly or indirectly to this population interchange. A significant proportion of Negro and Puerto Rican families are found at or close to the bottom of the income distribution. In 1966, New York State established an eligibility requirement for Medicaid of an income of $6,000 or less for a family of four. At peak before the 1968 cutback, city enrollment had reached 2.4 million. There is no firm basis for calculating the potential eligibles, but the total Medicaid population, enrolled and enrollable, probably amounted to between 40 and 50 percent of the city's population, with a heavy overrepresentation of minority groups. This is the first critical parameter. A high proportion, circa 50 percent, of New York City's population had to look to government for assistance in meeting some or all of its medical care costs.

In 1948–49, the expenditure budget of New York City amounted to $1.151 billion or roughly $150 per person. The budget for 1968-69 amounted to $5.994 billion or $750 per person. Even if we make a liberal allowance for the decline in the purchasing power of the dollar, circa 45 percent, the adjusted figures show a steep rise during these twenty years in both total and per capita governmental expenditures.

Against this background of rapidly rising municipal expenditures, the health and hospital operating budget of New York City climbed from $80 million in the late 1940s to $616 million in the late 1960s, and to a total municipal expenditure of $885 million including Medicaid. After adjusting for the 100 percent rise in the medical care price index for the New York area, this represents an increase in annual per capita municipal health expenditures, exclusive of Medicaid, from $10 to $38.

These few figures underscore the substantial increases in expenditures of municipal government during the past two decades, with a greater relative increase in expenditures for health and hospital care; widespread public dissatisfaction with the quality of municipal services, including health and medical care, cannot then be explained by frozen budgets. It is easy to contend, as many organizations have, that the City of New York has been remiss in not spending more money, since its budget has not been sufficient to provide quality services and an attractive environment. But these groups fail to take into account the constraints upon the city legislators when they attempt to raise tax rates. Higher tax rates will at some point become counterproductive since more businesses will relocate and thus produce a smaller tax base.

The population reshuffle that has dominated the last two decades has effected a vastly enhanced demand for a great variety of municipal services, including health and hospital care, and at the same time it has confronted the city with the necessity of raising the required taxes from a population which is continuing to lose middle- and upper-income families to the suburbs.

The population reshuffle had a second important impact on the demand and supply of medical services. Many neighborhoods, especially in Manhattan, Bronx, and Brooklyn, underwent radical transformations as whites moved out and minority groups moved in. As Professor Hiestand makes clear in the next chapter, New York City has a pluralistic health structure in which the private, non-profit, and governmental sectors all provide essential services. Voluntary hospitals, primarily under secular or sectarian control, used to provide for the ambulatory and inpatient needs of low-income families in established neighborhoods. They were able to do this in part by appointing to their staffs physicians who lived in the area or close by. These physicians were willing to contribute their services to poor patients on the wards and in the outpatient clinics in return for the privilege of admitting their private patients to the hospital and for the advantages that accrue from having a staff appointment. Prior to World War II physicians also sought appointments on the staffs of municipal hospitals where they contributed many hours of unpaid service in return for certain professional preferments such as participating in the hospital practice of medicine, the possibility of becoming a chief of service, and increasing their exposure to potential private patients.

But, as Mrs. Ostow points out in her analysis of affiliation contracts, much changed when the middle- and lower-income white families left and Negroes and Puerto Ricans moved in. Specifically, residency training came to be centered in the voluntary sector, making staff appointments in municipal hospitals less attractive. The demand for physicians' services from fee-paying patients rose so that many practitioners were disinclined to devote many hours to free hospital service. Finally the demographic shifts made it less likely for a physician on a municipal hospital staff to add to his potential clientele. In recent years the city has had to provide for an even larger proportion of the total medical needs of the low-income population. The participation of the voluntary sector has declined significantly.

We see, then, that knowledge of the population reshuffling which took place in New York City during the 1950s and 1960s is basic for understanding and evaluating the changes in the demand for, and supply of, municipal services, including education, social welfare, police, sanitation, and health. Attention must also be directed to developments more closely linked to the production of medical services if the points of challenge and response are to be seen in perspective. On the medical front the following trends are noteworthy.

The rapid expansion of Blue Cross and commercial insurance for inpatient hospital care made it possible for most voluntary hospitals to operate in the black, once they convinced the city to raise its reimbursement rates for welfare cases to a figure approximating their per diem costs. With the introduction of Medicare and Medicaid in 1966 the voluntary hospitals had an important new infusion of revenue which made it possible for them to meet at least some of the mounting pressures for higher wages and salaries from their non-professional and professional personnel. The new legislation also gave important assistance to the municipal hospital system, which had likewise been faced with demands for higher wages and salaries and improvements in working conditions, of which the city had been earlier able to meet only a small part. The fact that the federal and state governments found it necessary to cut back their appropriations for Medicaid within a few years left both the voluntary and the municipal hospitals in a vulnerable position, since both had raised their operating costs in anticipation of permanent new sources of income.

The last two decades have seen more and more medical service centered in the hospital. At the same time, the large university-based or -affiliated hospital has assumed a more important role as an educational and training institution. These trends have led to severe and continuing manpower pressures. Mr. Brecher sets forth the adjustments that took place in the educational and training structures in New York City in response to the large and continuing demand for more medical manpower. While expanded training of the allied health professions never caught up with the demand—in part because of the losses from the field that occurred because of unsatisfactory wages and working conditions—it did keep most personnel shortages within bounds.

The major exception was in attracting and retaining adequate house staff in municipal hospitals. Since, in an era of specialization, young medical school graduates opted for internships and residencies in hospitals that could offer strong training programs and since the municipal hospitals were unable to provide such programs, among other reasons because of a lack of full-time chiefs of service, the municipal system faced a major crisis at the beginning of the 1960s. The response to this physician crisis took the form of affiliation contracts between municipal and strong voluntary hospitals, a story that is told and interpreted by Mrs. Ostow in chapter 5.

The major problems that arose and the partial solutions that were developed centered on money and manpower. The third important dimension of medical care involves capital plant. The several aspects of this problem—new construction, maintenance, renovation—which relate to both the voluntary and the municipal system are reviewed in the chapters by Professors Greenfield and Yavitz. Professor Greenfield reviews the flow of funds, voluntary and public, that became available during these years to expand and improve hospital plant and calls attention to forces that influenced the size and distribution of this capital. He notes in particular the role of the quasi-public body—the Health and Hospital Planning Council of Southern New York, Inc.—which under state legislation has been given certain broad planning and allocative responsibilities.

Professor Yavitz's chapter is concerned with the city's capital budgeting process, from proposal to completion of a hospital project. The New York City Health and Hospitals Corporation, with a sixteen-member board, was recently authorized by the state legislature to provide a more flexible mechanism for operating the city's municipal hospitals and for overseeing maintenance and new construction. It has been generally acknowledged that unless a new agency with some freedom from the plethora of bureaucratic rules and regulations in decision-making were established, the municipal system would not be able to improve the quality of its operations. It remains to be seen how effective the new device will be; if the available resources are grossly inadequate, its chief challenge will be optimal allocation and utilization of the funds at its disposal.

One of the interesting adaptations that occurred in recent years in the pattern of medical care in New York City relates to the rapid expansion of emergency room services, a development reviewed here and appraised by Professor Zubkoff. This innovation is interesting particularly because it occurred largely in response to consumer pressure with relatively little or no formal planning by the hospitals. In the face of a shortage of physician manpower, worst in the low-income areas of the city, more and more people who needed medical attention went to the emergency room of a hospital in their immediate or adjacent neighborhood. Often they were encouraged to do so by busy practitioners who were unable or unwilling to make house calls. Even today most hospitals with emergency rooms have not yet decided how best to staff and operate them. Moreover, as Professor Zubkoff makes clear, few hospitals have taken the additional important step of developing a rational payment scheme for emergency services.

Although emergency services expanded substantially over the past decade, ambulatory services experienced relatively modest changes, as Mr. Brecher and Mrs. Ostow indicate in their analysis. Outpatient services remained relatively static despite the rapidly rising costs of inpatient care and despite the repeated urgings by leaders of the medical profession to broaden the scope of ambulatory care. Apparently the combined impact of insurance systems that defensively continued to limit coverage primarily to inpatients, the absence of hospital-based group practice units, the inability or lack of desire of hospitals to modernize and rationalize their ambulatory services, and recently the encouragement that Medicaid has given the poor to patronize private physicians, has been to retard experimentation and expansion of strong ambulatory services. A few interesting efforts with city funds were made initially at Gouverneur Hospital, followed by the establishment of several neighborhood health centers supported by federal grants chiefly from the Office of Economic Opportunity. While definitive evaluations have not yet been made, our colleagues have reservations about the potential of these experiments to replicate themselves. The per capita costs are high and consumers' benefits are more often than not found in areas tangential to health care—for instance, in local employment and in political organization.

Although much has been written about the desirability of introducing regional planning in the health system to ensure a more economical and efficient allocation and distribution of scarce resources, the simple fact is that relatively little progress has been made, nationally or locally.

Mr. Brecher's chapter on the limited regionalization which has developed in the borough of the Bronx provides an interesting case example of a desirable but little-implemented objective in hospital and medical planning. The story that he unravels points to the many preconditions for progress: institutional interest, strong professional leadership, the availability of funds for new developments, and the absence of entrenched political and professional opposition to change. Small wonder that successful efforts are the exception. Much more than logic is needed to bring a regional effort to fruition.

The final substantive chapter provides more information about the potentialities of and resistances to change. In reviewing what happened and what failed to happen as a consequence of the early 1950 breakthrough in the chemotherapeutic treatment of tuberculosis, Mrs. Ostow shows the great difficulties athwart any attempt to modify existing institutions and practices, even when the system is presented with an opportunity to shift the focus of therapy from prolonged bed rest to ambulatory treatment. Her analysis further records the urgent need for leaders of the medical profession to realize that for improved therapy for diseases such as tuberculosis, and in the pursuit of public health objectives generally, effective programs must go beyond the purely medical. Many patients, current and potential, will not be reached or treated unless the community can be encouraged to play a role and unless new types of personnel can be trained and utilized to carry most of the responsibility for bringing the poor and alienated into the medical system and for helping to monitor their treatment.

So much for the discrete aspects of the changing medical scene to which this book is responsive. It was never our intent to provide an inclusive view of recent developments in urban medical care. That would have been beyond our resources and would not have served our central purpose. For instance, it would have been interesting and revealing to include a chapter on child health and maternal services, both to emphasize the gains that have been made and the reasons for them and to point up the persistent deficiencies and the obstacles to further advances. The efforts to expand and improve mental health services would likewise have provided an important case study of new efforts that combine limited success with many failures.

These and other important dimensions of the medical care system have not been included because this book by design did not aim at a comprehensive review and assessment of the quantity and quality of medical services available to the population of New York City. Its focus is narrower and more specific. We sought to explore in some depth selected dimensions of urban health services and thus to uncover the forces leading to change and those which stop or retard change. Our primary concern was to deepen understanding of a pluralistic decision-making process in which no group, not even municipal government with annual operating expenditures of $885 million (1969), has significant leverage on the redesign and production of medical services.

At the heart of our concern are such questions as these: To what extent can changes be made in the production and distribution of health services if a key group such as physicians or voluntary hospitals is opposed to change? How potent a force for change are additional dollar expenditures in the face of a substantially inelastic supply of trained manpower? What were the payoffs—and to whom —from the several hundred million dollars that became available as a result of Medicaid?

Since services depend in the first instance on the availability of trained manpower, how can a democratic society such as ours ensure that the educational-training structures are kept in step with the expanded requirements for additional professional and allied personnel? How is access to essential services ensured in a society such as ours characterized by substantial inequality of income, discrimination, concentration of poor people in particular neighborhoods? Since these differences exist, is it sensible to promise that everybody is entitled to quality services? What meaning does such a concept have?

Since the nongovernmental sector is responsible for the management of general hospitals which primarily cater to the needs of paying patients, what leverage does New York City have to ensure that it is not permanently saddled with two hospital systems—one for the paying, one for the indigent population? In the absence of effective leverage to alter this stand-off relation, what can the city do to keep its commitments in bounds and to provide a reasonable quality of service for those for whom it is responsible?

New York City is faced with two critically important new developments: the rapid unionization of municipal workers and the mounting pressure for decentralization of planning and operating control over municipal services to various community groups throughout the five boroughs. How can the city determine on an equitable wage among its competing labor groups and, further, how can it ensure that the wage structures are kept in balance with the consumers' and taxpayers' willingness and ability to pay? Moreover, what policies can the city pursue to be responsive to the legitimate claims for community participation while preserving a significant role for centralized professional leadership?

We have explored these complex issues. More often than not, our explanations stop short of definitive judgments and recommendations. Yet our analyses have enabled us to obtain new and better information about the provision of urban health services. And by presenting new perspectives on this one service, the book helps to open up a series of related problems germane to the gamut of urban services in a pluralistic society.

1

PLURALISM
IN HEALTH SERVICES

THIS CHAPTER will delineate the pluralistic nature of the health services complex within New York City and the implications of this for public policy. "Pluralism" is a word which is increasingly used; therefore, we must make clear the kind of pluralism to which we refer. We are primarily concerned with the pluralism of the economic and managerial aspects of health services. Since this involves the determination and execution of policy, we are also concerned with political pluralism as it operates overtly through the governmental apparatus and throughout the various institutions, enterprises, and groups which make up the health services complex.

Pluralism is the division of position, power, responsibility, or obligation among groups or institutions; it implies both sharing and competition, frequently conflict, although it does not imply hostility.

In considering health services we must understand their pluralistic nature, which results from three unique aspects:

1. Health services are provided through diverse institutional forms (private enterprises, nonprofit enterprises, and government agencies) which are responsive to many different groups and agencies.

2. Payments for health services are made by a broad range of purchasers: the individual consumer, profit-seeking and not-for-profit enterprises, philanthropic organizations, foundations, and government.

3. Inputs of resources to the health services complex come from a variety of institutions which operate under a complicated system of control and influence. Pluralism is particularly operative in the

development of manpower for the health services and in the accumulation of capital funds for building and equipment.

The recent increase in pluralism is not confined to the health services sector. Rather, pluralism seems to be a generalized trend in the production of goods and services in the United States, conspicuously in the areas of defense, space, and education. Health services are unique, however, in the pervasiveness of pluralism with respect to production, financing, and manpower. In contrast, the federal government is the only customer for defense and space. Again in contrast, a distinct part of the educational system, the parochial schools, has not received much direct financial support from public funds.

The managerial and political implications of pluralism in the health services complex are important. As we shall see, since responsibility for individual aspects of the system is usually shared, cooperation is necessary if the system is to perform effectively. With many different groups and interests enjoying positions of power and influence, agreement, or at least the absence of hostility, is a precondition for sound action. Moreover, since so much of the delivery of inputs and the purchase of services involves government, agreement may be contractual, political, or administrative in form, or any combination of these.

PLURALISM IN THE PROVISION
OF SERVICES

The most obvious type of pluralism is evidenced in the institutional forms into which health services enterprises in New York City are organized. As Table 1.1 indicates, most hospitals in the city are operated by voluntary nonprofit organizations, which have more beds and patients than hospitals of any other institutional form. These voluntary hospitals provide general care, including medical, surgical, pediatric, and maternity services.

Municipal hospitals, next largest in terms of total bed complement, also provide primarily general care, although one-fourth of their beds and of their average daily census are devoted to long-term care. The state hospitals, which are mental hospitals, actually

TABLE 1.1

*Number, Bed Complement, and Average Daily Census
of Hospitals in New York City, by Type*

Type	No. of Hospitals 1/1/68	Bed Complement 1/1/68	Average Daily Census 1967
Voluntary	80	26,933	23,524
Local government	18	17,013	13,491
Proprietary	36	4,827	4,082
State	6	14,921	14,357
Federal	5	5,395	4,667
Total	145	69,089	60,121

Source: Health and Hospital Planning Council of Southern New York, Inc.

have an average daily census which exceeds that of the municipal hospitals. There are a great number of proprietary or privately owned hospitals, but they account for only 7 percent of all beds and inpatients. The five federal hospitals (three Veterans Administration hospitals, one Naval hospital, and one Public Health Service hospital) have a larger bed capacity and average census than all the private hospitals combined.

This tabulation does not include nursing homes, though a small number of nursing care beds are included in a few of the hospitals. As Table 1.2 indicates, the large majority of nursing facilities are privately owned and operated. Most of the voluntary nursing-home care is provided in the infirmaries of homes for the aged; the

TABLE 1.2

Nursing Home Facilities in New York City, by Type

Type	Number of Facilities 1/1/68	Number of Beds 1/1/68
Voluntary	52	4,904
Local government	5	1,956
Proprietary	92	11,622
Total	149	18,482

Source: Health and Hospital Planning Council of Southern New York, Inc.

balance is divided among nursing homes, special units in hospitals, and convalescent homes. A small number of extended care facilities are found in special units of municipal hospitals.

Health facilities in New York City cannot be considered in isolation, since they serve people from the suburbs and beyond, while city residents who want care may go outside. In 1966, for instance, 9 percent of the New York City residents receiving chronic care in the Southern New York Region were in institutions outside the city. On the other hand, some 2 percent of all the patients of facilities in the city were from the suburban counties.

Let us turn from institutions to services. The initial contact for services made by patients is usually the physician in private practice. He may practice alone or in a partnership. A significant number of physicians in New York are partners or employees of prepaid group schemes such as HIP (Health Insurance Plan of Greater New York). Recently, as a later chapter shows, the initial contact with a physician is increasingly made in a hospital emergency room, even when a patient has a minor complaint. Care is also provided by a great variety of hospital-operated clinics.

The services available from the physician of initial contact depend on his situation and that of the patient. Physicians vary greatly with regard to the kinds of cases they treat and this fact determines their diagnostic and therapeutic equipment and the types of personnel they employ.

If outside diagnostic or therapeutic services are required, the physician may utilize or refer the patient to hospital facilities, privately operated laboratories, independent health agencies, public services, independent medical or allied practitioners, and the like. If he lacks a hospital staff appointment or is faced with a case that is too difficult or not in his preferred area of work, the physician may refer his patient to a colleague, frequently a specialist.

Once the patient is in the hospital, the full mix of hospital resources, both manpower and equipment, can be brought to work on his behalf. The pluralistic nature of the situation is crucial here, for the physician in private practice is enabled to utilize and in effect direct the employees and facilities of the hospital in the care of his patients. After the patient has been discharged, he may continue to be served by the hospital's home care service. Some patients may periodically receive care at home from various public or voluntary health services.

In the hospital setting, the physician is subject to the collegial relations within the staff. Various forms of restrictions and review procedures inhibit or influence his actions. From the physician's point of view, these procedures have positive value: they protect as well as instruct him and potentially enhance his professional status. To provide the necessary professional and financial preconditions for staff sufficiency and stability, a series of affiliation agreements have been reached between various medical schools and voluntary hospitals, on the one hand, and the municipal hospital system, on the other. Under the terms of these agreements, which are extensively considered in a later chapter, the affiliate provides all professional and some technical staff to the related municipal facility; the result has been a remarkable increase in the recruiting strength of the municipal hospitals particularly for residents and interns. The wider effect has been to intermingle greatly the affairs of voluntary and municipal hospitals, and to extend the influence of voluntary leadership upon public policy and expenditures. City subsidization of the voluntary hospitals has increased significantly, and the city's position has shifted from producer to purchaser of in-hospital professional services.

In another development, the city has arranged for a voluntary hospital to assume complete operation of a municipal facility: since 1969 the James Ewing Hospital has been leased to Memorial Hospital.

Hospital affiliations and leasing have been one step in the changing relations of public and private health services producers. As of mid-1970, management, capital construction, and maintenance of the city's hospital plant has been transferred to the New York City Health and Hospitals Corporation, a public-benefit corporation directed by mandated municipal officials and appointed private citizens. This marks the end of direct operation of hospitals by the city but not the end of direct fiscal responsibility.

Finally, the city's Department of Hospitals has also been responsible for licensing and inspecting proprietary hospitals and nursing homes. Thus the city has a direct influence on both existing and contemplated operations in the private sector.

The pluralistic nature of the health services complex continues to be evident when we consider how services are paid for. This section is concerned with the financing of operating services; the next section, with capital financing.

It is difficult to delineate precisely the various money flows for current services into this complex, but the general nature of the system is clear. Direct payments by the individual consumer are less common than is payment by some intermediate agency. Perhaps two-thirds of the population of New York City are covered by some form of hospital insurance, and a somewhat smaller proportion is insured for physicians' services. The majority of the remaining third are covered by Medicare or Medicaid.

Hospitalization insurance may be in the form of a group or individual contract with Blue Cross or with a mutual or stock insurance company; analogous coverage for physicians' services may be provided by Blue Shield, a commercial insurance company, GHI (Group Health Insurance, Inc.), HIP, or some other group plan. Insurance coverages vary according to whether they reimburse the consumer or the provider for services rendered. More significant variation is found in the scope and extent of benefits: in-hospital or ambulatory services, diagnostic or therapeutic care, ancillary requirements, etc.

Medicare is, of course, a form of insurance federally required and carried in a special fund of the Social Security Administration. Medicaid is technically a local program, although it operates under state and federal laws, with intergovernmental financing. The city pays about 30 percent of the costs, the state 30 percent, and the federal government 40 percent.

Approximately 15 percent of the New York City Executive Budget goes for health services. In fiscal 1968–69, for instance, appropriations for health services came to $884.8 million out of a total executive budget of $6,006.6 million. As Table 1.3 indicates, nearly half of this budget was for the municipal hospital system, and nearly one-third for Medicaid payments to private practitioners, private hospitals, and voluntary hospitals. State and federal cost-sharing in Medicaid also reimburses the city for services to eligible patients in the municipal hospitals.

These payments systems have other, more important pluralistic aspects. Most group insurance plans are organized through places of employment. Often, employers pay part or all of the premiums. For blue-collar workers and public employees, the terms of the insurance coverage and the method of payment are usually part

TABLE 1.3

Health Services Appropriations, City of New York, 1968–1969
(in millions of dollars)

Municipal hospital care	$421.5
Payments to voluntary hospitals for inpatient care of Medicaid eligibles	85.3
Payments to private practitioners and institutions for services provided Medicaid eligibles	196.0
Public health	64.5
Mental health	111.9
Other	5.6
Total	$884.8

Source: City of New York, Executive Budget, 1969–70.

of collective bargaining agreements. Blue Cross and Blue Shield are organized by the hospitals and the medical societies respectively. HIP and GHI were designed primarily to serve public employees, particularly city employees, and trade unions, which means that union and public officials are centrally involved in their operations and policy determination. More recently some unions and employers have also taken a direct interest in Blue Cross and Blue Shield operations.

Blue Cross plays a critical role through its function of reimbursing hospitals on a per diem basis for treating enrolled patients, a mode of payment which has been carried over into the Medicare and Medicaid programs. On the other hand, commercial insurance companies and Blue Shield tend to pay all or part of the charges incurred by the recipients of services. In either case the determination of allowable expenses or charges becomes a highly important matter for all concerned. The establishment of criteria or definitions, of methods of validation and verification, regularly involves much controversy, negotiation, and political settlement.

In the past the commercial insurance companies and the employers and unions which use them have played a passive role with respect to operations and policies affecting either expenses or services. For the entire range of nonprofit and commercial plans, rate schedules must be approved by the New York State Insurance Commission. This procedure involves public hearings as well as *in camera* negotiations on all possible determinants of cost and sound fiscal practice. The political process dictates a key role for commissioners, staff personnel, and the like. Members of the legislature and elected officials are intimately involved in legislation, appointments, and appropriations affecting the Insurance Commission, the State Health Department, and other concerned agencies and their policy-making apparatus. Recently, the mayor of the City of New York, the controller, and ultimately the state courts interposed themselves (unsuccessfully) between the consumer public and the State Insurance Commission in response to a very large premium revision.

The Medicaid program has had diverse impacts on the city's health system. It has provided additional federal and state funds to supplement and substitute for city tax revenues. However, the free choice given the indigent has led to a diversion of much of this new stream of funds into the voluntary and private hospitals, as well as into the hands of private practitioners. With additional funds flowing into voluntary, private, and governmental institutions, the competition for manpower and other resources has accelerated and the struggle for salary increases has intensified, particularly at the top and bottom of the scale. The voluntary and proprietary systems, having greater flexibility with respect to wages and personnel practices, increased their wages rapidly, an action that was reflected before long in the contracts of affiliated municipal hospitals. The promise of continuing Medicaid funds also stimulated the city to undertake an ambitious innovative program, a network of family ambulatory care centers. With the Medicaid cutbacks in 1969, instability and uncertainty of income has unsettled both sectors. The voluntary institutions have been embarrassed by their much higher cost levels. And the city has been burdened with complete responsibility for about a million patients formerly eligible for Medicaid.

PLURALISM IN OBTAINING
CAPITAL RESOURCES

For over two decades, the federal Hill-Burton program has stimulated the accumulation and utilization of capital funds for health facilities. Conceived by Congress for the purpose of improving the nation's health plant, seriously deficient after almost twenty years of depression and war, the Hill-Burton program has granted funds to the states for facilities construction, equipment, and rehabilitation.

Initially, Congress specified that monies be made available primarily to areas lacking hospital and health facilities, mainly rural and sparsely settled areas; since 1964, priority has shifted to the modernization of older hospitals in urban areas.

The states have considerable option with regard to how the funds will be allocated geographically and among the different classes and types of facilities. For each project the public or nonprofit sponsoring agency is required to raise independently a minimum of two-thirds of the cost.

The allocation of federal funds must be in accordance with a comprehensive state plan which defines needs and establishes programs to meet these needs. In New York, the plan is prepared each year by the Division of Hospital Review and Planning of the State Health Department, which depends in turn on the recommendations of a series of regional hospital and health facilities planning agencies. The Health and Hospital Planning Council of Southern New York, Inc., a nonprofit organization, serves New York City and nine downstate counties.

The individual planning agencies must also reach policy decisions involving geographic units, sponsoring groups, types of facilities, and preferred types of construction. Their choices with respect to different technical criteria inevitably affect a great many interest groups.

To a considerable extent, a wide range of agencies and groups with different objectives and constituencies are directly involved in the policy-determining process. Represented within the Health and Hospital Planning Council of Southern New York are sectarian charitable agencies, trade unions, hospital and nursing home associations, medical societies, business associations, voluntary health and welfare agencies, and Blue Cross, a total of twenty-five organizations. The Council's board of directors includes in addition private citizens and public officials, and it depends heavily on a variety of committees with members drawn both from within and without the board.

As noted earlier, the program initially favored rural and outlying areas. In New York City, Hill-Burton funds constituted a smaller proportion of total project cost or even of the total cost of projects eligible for such funds than elsewhere. Between 1948 and 1963, less than half the costs of projects in the city were eligible to be considered for Hill-Burton aid, compared to 83 percent in the rest of the region.

More recent figures suggest that the city still gets a relatively small share of federal hospital construction funds. Between 1961 and 1966, for instance, the city received 13 percent of all federal funds granted to New York State for the construction of hospital and medical facilities. However, New York City received a considerably bigger share, about 40 percent, of all federal grants for other facilities, including those for health and mental retardation research, health teaching, and community mental health centers. Over half of these funds were allocated for health research facilities, and they went largely to the seven medical schools.

In the final analysis, the Hill-Burton funds are the smallest part of capital funds raised for health facilities in the city. The various voluntary groups, including religious and charitable organizations, and the municipal and state governments are the primary media through which capital funds are accumulated.

The growth of pluralistic payment mechanisms is tending to have an effect on the method of financing health facilities. Increasingly, depreciation and the cost of capital are included as allowable expenses within private and public systems of hospital insurance. This makes it possible for organizations to borrow capital funds and repay the debt out of future income.

PLURALISM IN THE

DEVELOPMENT AND UTILIZATION

OF HEALTH MANPOWER

The manpower component of the health services sector includes a broad range of occupations from the most highly skilled to the unskilled. A complex system of specialized and general institutions is involved in the training of the different occupational groups. Recently a major effort was started to upgrade even the most unskilled of these workers.

Physicians, of course, are trained in the medical schools and teaching hospitals. There are at the present time seven medical schools in New York City. Internships are offered by sixty-one hospitals, and residencies by eighty-two hospitals in the city.

There is also an active program of continuing medical education; four nonprofit schools in the city offer accredited programs to practicing physicians. Other training at the doctoral level is limited. Two universities operate dental schools and there is one private school of podiatry. In addition, a wide variety of programs for allied health professionals—hospital administrators, rehabilitation counselors, sanitary engineers, pharmacists, dietitians, health educators, medical librarians, occupational and physical therapists, psychologists, and medical technologists—is offered by the nonprofit and public colleges and universities in the city. The arena of allied health manpower, which has undergone significant expansion in the last decade, is treated more extensively by Mr. Charles Brecher in the next chapter.

The large majority of nurses are trained in hospital schools of nursing. But there is a definite trend toward training nurses in associate degree programs in collegiate institutions. The smallest group are those trained in bachelor's degree programs. Schools of nursing are operated by three state, four municipal, and nineteen voluntary hospitals in New York City. Associate degree programs are available at seven community colleges in the City University of New York. There are nine college and university baccalaureate programs, six in private universities and three in the City University.

The system is still more complex. To furnish an adequate range of clinical experiences to their students, the large majority of schools, even the hospital schools of nursing, utilize two or more hospitals. In these programs, faculty members may accompany their students into the host facility to provide supervision. More than one facility is used when the home hospital does not include a full range of specialized services, or if it is a specialized institution and its students need general medical-surgical experience. The most extensive network of clinical relationships is that of the program at Queens College, which places its students at Booth Memorial, Flushing, Francis Delafield, Hillside, and Long Island Jewish hospitals, and at the Queens Hospital Center. There is no necessary connection between the sponsorship of the schools and the hospitals: voluntary, municipal, and state institutions in the city and the suburbs collaborate freely. In addition, a few hospital schools of nursing rely on nearby junior or senior colleges to teach the basic sciences to their students. The baccalaureate programs also provide for periods of public health service with the Visiting Nurse Service of New York, the Visiting Nurse Association of Brooklyn, and the Public Health Division of the New York City Department of Health.

Community colleges play an increasing role in the training of personnel for the health services in the city. In addition to nursing, they offer programs for a variety of medical and laboratory technicians and other health occupations. Many of these programs are run cooperatively with the Department of Hospitals, District Council No. 37 of the American Federation of State, County, and Municipal Employees, and the U.S. Department of Labor. In 1968, for instance, some 1,900 municipal hospital employees were enrolled in such joint programs to qualify for advancement, as from nurse's aide to practical nurse.

The U.S. Department of Labor has been active in promoting allied health training in the community colleges to upgrade employees of both municipal and voluntary hospitals; it has also supported on-the-job training within the hospitals. Most of these programs are directed to licensed practical nurses and nurse's aides. In addition, the public vocational schools offer training to nurse's aides, orderlies, and practical nurses.

While the range of health training facilities has been described for each occupational level independently, in point of fact the various curricula are organizationally related. The Columbia University health education complex, for instance, includes a medical school, school of public health and administrative medicine, dental school, nursing school, graduate nursing education department, and pharmacy school. It also has affiliation agreements with two municipal hospitals. Its nursing departments use voluntary and municipal hospitals and public health agencies for clinical experience. It also operates municipal clinics and has a student health service in St. Luke's Medical Center, a voluntary hospital.

Similarly, the City University is organizing a health professions complex involving a private nonprofit medical school, the Mount Sinai School of Medicine, the Hunter College Institute of Health Sciences, and a new Community College for Health Careers. This complex will utilize a wide variety of voluntary and governmental hospitals for clinical training. There will also be some coordination with the health training programs in the other junior and senior colleges of the City University.

The accreditation of schools and state licensing provisions play an important role in determining the number as well as the quality of those who are trained. To establish or enlarge a medical school, approval of the Association of American Medical Colleges and the American Medical Association is required; the latter also accredits internships and residencies. Educational programs, as well as licensing provisions, also require the approval of the State Board of Regents, which relies upon recommendations of professional committees. Dentistry is similarly organized.

The National League for Nursing is the recognized accrediting agency for nursing schools. Accreditation is not necessary, however, and half of all programs in the state are unaccredited. As far as licensure is concerned, organized nursing is influential but not controlling. The associations of practical nurses and technicians play an even less crucial role in the approval of schools and licensure provisions affecting their occupations. For some purposes, the medical profession is, in fact, more influential than the nursing and other allied health associations in determining the details of training and licensure in their respective occupations.

The financing of health manpower educational programs taps multiple streams. The Public Health Training Act of 1960, the Health Professions Educational Assistance Act of 1963, the Nurse Training Act of 1964, the Allied Health Professions Personnel Training Act of 1966, the Health Manpower Act of 1968, and the Higher Education Act variously provide funds for construction and renovation of health educational facilities, teaching grants, and student financial aid. In addition, New York State provides money independently and on a matching basis for such purposes. From the point of view of the total finances of medical schools, the wide range of research grants from the National Institutes of Health and other federal agencies, plus grants under the Health Research Facilities Act of 1966 and the Mental Retardation Facilities and Community Mental Health Centers Construction Act of 1963, has been far more influential than educational grants.

For nonprofessional levels, the importance of Manpower Development and Training Act funds, which support the programs in which the U.S. Department of Labor is involved, should be noted. Similarly, allied health training in the vocational high schools receives significant federal financial support.

While hospitals operating training schools may have some advantage in subsequently hiring those they train, their graduates and those of junior and senior colleges are free to seek employment where they will. There is no necessary connection between the sector or even the geographical area in which a person is trained and where he is ultimately employed. Most nurses are employed in hospitals, but more than one-third work in other health services.

The interaction of manpower supply and relative pay scales affects the distribution of personnel among hospitals. At the level of nurse's aides and below, hospitals tend to have relatively low wage rates, and differentials among institutions are minor and have little effect. For such unskilled workers, each hospital is able to recruit from the immediate neighborhood or from low-income neighborhoods along a convenient subway or bus route. At the level of technician, nurse, secretary, craftsman and above, hospitals may find it necessary to recruit over a wider area in the city or in the suburbs, and in the case of nurses, they have even gone abroad. In such cases, wage differentials can have a significant effect.

Historically, there have been persistent differentials between voluntary and municipal hospital salary scales for higher-level workers. There is evidence that voluntary hospital administrators seek to avoid competition with each other, and city officials charged with adjusting municipal salary schedules may also avoid aggressive competition with philanthropic agencies. The maintenance of a lower salary schedule in the municipal hospital system, even during a period of inflation, reflects the historic difficulties of adjusting public pay scales to the market.

The result has been that a far higher proportion of budgeted positions in municipal hospitals has been vacant. Within the last few years, however, salary increases in the public service have tended to reduce the salary differentials. As a result, the proportion of vacancies among nursing, technician, and similar positions has also tended to decline.

The important point within the present context is not so much the differentials in salaries and vacancies as the fact that salary schedules in the various systems seem not to have been determined independently. The voluntary hospitals are directly concerned when municipal hospital salary schedules are raised, but since they retain more flexibility to adjust to market changes they tend to be better staffed, are able to provide a more generally adequate level of nursing and technical services, and are consequently more attractive to physicians and patients.

EMERGING FORMS OF PLURALISM

Given the rapid growth of the health services sector, it is to be expected that many problems will emerge. Characteristically, the proposals for dealing with pressing problems almost invariably include an expansion in the degree and forms of pluralism. Generally, progress is sought by changing some of the relationships among different parts of the system, but its pluralistic nature is maintained. A case in point is the recent establishment of a Health and Hospitals Corporation to operate the municipal hospital system. Hospital policy, however, will continue to be fixed by the Health Services Administration.

One issue which continues to reappear is how the consumers of health services can have any influence on the health services complex. As the complex is currently constituted, effective power tends to lie with the groups and institutions producing services; secondary power, largely unused, resides with those agencies and institutions which supply funds. With prevailing shortages of physicians and hospital beds, however, the consumer has a limited choice, whether or not he pays his bill personally. If, in addition, various payment mechanisms are linked to specific producers or create strong incentives toward their use, the consumer has even less influence.

To some degree, consumer interests are considered by the various groups and institutions which do affect the health complex, particularly the legislature and governmental agencies charged with determination of the "public interest." But inevitably the producer interest has been more effectively represented along with the governmental, that is, bureaucratic, interest.

In an attempt to involve the consumer more directly, Congress provided in 1966 (Public Law 89-749) for funds to stimulate the organization in various jurisdictions of comprehensive health-planning agencies which would represent more equitably producers, consumers, and government. The organization of such agencies has turned out to be an extremely difficult political problem. In the City of New York there was a complete stalemate for over two years; after vehement controversy the city was authorized by the state in the spring of 1969 to designate an Organizational Task Force which would in turn generate a planning agency. This initial body of fifty-seven members was named in October, 1969, by the mayor. Its composition is perhaps the best example of how pluralistic the health services complex already is. The twenty-nine consumer members represent neighborhood-based and city-wide consumer groups, the New York City Council Against Poverty, the mayor, the City Planning Commission, the City Council, regional planning organizations, commerce and industry, labor, older people, groups concerned with environmental health, mental health and retardation, and education, and each of the boroughs. The twenty-eight producers' representatives have as their constituencies voluntary and private hospitals and nursing homes, home care agencies, the Health and Hospital Planning Council of Southern New York, health insurance organizations, medical societies, dental societies, nursing organizations, other allied health professional groups, mental health practitioners, the Health Services Administration, the Environmental Protection Administration, the Human Resources Administration, and the Regional Medical Program in New York City. The evolution of an effective planning agency and planning process from this task force suggests the labors of Sisyphus.

Municipal and voluntary hospitals have traditionally involved community groups in voluntary and auxiliary services such as operating or equipping gift shops, beauty parlors, playrooms, and employee facilities, as well as providing direct service (frequently recreational or social) to patients.

Recently more important and far-reaching departures have developed in the involvement of community groups. Significantly, the New York Health and Hospitals Corporation has been legally empowered to contract with subsidiary local operating bodies for health facilities under its jurisdiction. This reflects the ideological thrust of the Piel Report (1967) toward decentralization of city health services and an explicit degree of community planning and review. But such a step is well in the future: legislation restricts local subcontracting for a minimum of two years after the Corporation has commenced operations.

IMPLICATIONS OF PLURALISM IN
THE HEALTH SERVICES SECTOR

Perhaps the most important aspect of the elaboration of pluralism in the health services complex has to do with how growth and change can be accomplished. One can reasonably conclude that it is almost impossible for a single individual, institution, or group to effect any independent action. Decisions about new departures, new programs, even new buildings can only be made jointly, after all the different interests involved have been consulted and their differences mediated.

This phenomenon has further implications. Those who would exercise leadership must understand all the linkages involved in making any innovation. We have attempted here to lay out the nature of those linkages. We have not been able to indicate— because we really do not know—how much power and influence each of the interest groups has in each of the linkage systems. For effective leadership, one would have to understand these power relationships, and particularly areas of joint interest and antipathy.

The high order of pluralism which has been built into the health services complex may mean that there is a strong tendency toward the maintenance of the status quo. With many interest groups built into almost every decision system, each one tends to have a veto over any changes. These vetoes are likely to be exercised by any group which fears that a new departure may undermine or be adverse to its interests.

A further implication, therefore, is that innovations must almost inevitably be tailored so as not to threaten any interest groups and at the same time to provide positive incentives for the acquiescence, indeed the active support, of each of them.

As already suggested, we have only been able to outline the various relationships of power and influence at work in the health services complex. Much more needs to be known about the overt and, more importantly, the latent and emerging forms of control and leverage. In the larger sense, only as these relationships are understood will we know what is possible managerially.

The extent of pluralism in the health sector has led many to despair. Walter Reuther denied that the health services complex can be called a system. As he observed, "What we have, in fact, is a disorganized, disjointed, antiquated, obsolete, non-system of health care." The National Advisory Commission on Health Manpower has also asserted, "The word, 'system,' is . . . inaccurate if it implies the existence of an organized, coordinated, planned undertaking."

The health services complex is a system, however, but with goals beyond that of simply delivering health services. One basic goal, as the above discussion makes clear, is to protect the interests of the various groups involved in the production of these services. This goal, perhaps more than any other factor, accounts for the complexity of the pluralism in the health services sector.

CONCLUDING OBSERVATIONS

Charting the labyrinthine structure and relationships within which health services are produced in New York City would be merely an intellectual exercise if it yielded no significant insights for policy determination.

Critics of the existent system have attributed to its pluralism all the deficiencies of fragmentation, maldistribution, high cost, manpower shortages, overemphasis on therapy and underemphasis on prevention, that stand in the way of optimal application of an ever-increasing level of scientific knowledge and technical sophistication. As they see it, pluralism renders the system resistant to any but peripheral change because of the conflicting interests, goals, and priorities of its constituents. Hence, social welfare leaders have classically proposed that the two aspects of health care of immediate interest to the consumer, financing and delivery, must each be reorganized into a universal system through federal legislation. But without an apposite model for securing adequate inputs, reorganization of payment and delivery would not guarantee optimal change for the consumer. That consideration aside, however, it is apparent from our analysis that nowhere has sufficient leverage existed to effect such a sweeping systemic revision.

Yet it is precisely the area of financing that in the two past decades has undergone radical transformation through the massive development of voluntary insurance and the institution by the federal government of direct payment for care of specific segments of the civilian population, a commitment which was vastly extended by the Social Security legislation of 1965 (Medicare-Medicaid). Today, about 80 percent of the population have some form of medical insurance, and current proposals for universal national health insurance suggest a reorganization of existent structures rather than radical innovation. Identification of the diverse advocates of these proposals, spanning the leadership of organized labor and a score of Republican governors, makes this apparent.

Although it is not distinctly within the framework of municipal decision-making, this somewhat paradoxical development has been stressed because it reveals an essential aspect of the dynamics of pluralism: change, even basic change, occurs incrementally and is effected by political compromise and by shifting organizational alignments. A static model of conflicting interest groups and organizations able to nullify effective change through cross-veto is not valid, certainly not in the long run.

Within the city, there has been considerable movement over the past decade in the health system: structural, financial, and in terms of additional resources. Most dramatic, but not most efficacious, have been new and increased money flows, which at best have supported preexistent services without effecting enhancement or expansion; at worst they have inflated costs beyond the financial tolerances of the city. To a lesser extent, funds have underwritten innovative programs, whose value would be maximized through integration within the existent system and incorporation of their key features by the ongoing services. As opposed to the minimally productive new funding for services, there has been distinct enhancement in the quantity and quality of programs for allied health manpower training. It is significant that these programs have evolved as the result of new linkages between health and education systems in partial response to the needs of deprived urban populations.

For the city, the problem is not absence of change but lack of coordination and control over change, the result of limited planning capacity and effective leadership. To achieve satisfactory control would require a clear understanding of ongoing and emerging linkages as they impinge upon the health system, the hierarchy of interest groups in terms of the power they wield, and the succession of organizational alignments and realignments through which the political process asserts itself.

To effect planned change within the system requires leverage, of which the city has been woefully short. Money, however, is

potentially the most powerful lever of all. With increasing dependence of nonpublic health programs and institutions upon
public funds, and with the city serving as the generator or at least
the conduit for a major portion of these funds, municipal government has—if it wishes—the potential for the exercise of far greater
control and more effective planning capability than it has exercised
in the past. One key to the use of this capability is the priorities
that the mayor will establish for his administration.

2

EXPANDING MANPOWER RESOURCES

ONCE MEDICINE WAS exclusively the concern of physicians; today there are almost ten others employed in health services for each doctor. These others, currently referred to as "allied health manpower," are a mixture of individuals whose job preparation ranges from several days of on-the-job training to several years of post-college education. This wide range of training is provided at a variety of institutions including hospitals, universities, community colleges, and high schools. For some occupations, more than one institution provides the training. Practical nurses are trained at hospitals, high schools, and even, in New York City, at a YWCA; registered nurses are trained at colleges and hospitals. For other occupations one type of institution does the training. For example, a pharmacist can be licensed only after graduating from a five-year college program. The content and the duration of training for any one occupation are important to many groups, including those in the profession, those who employ them, those who must train them, and those who are served by them.

It is our purpose to extrapolate from this mixture of occupations, institutions, and interests the sources and directions of change which have been active in the last decade. Of equal importance are the patterns that have not changed and the attempted innovations which failed. Forces upholding the status quo are as significant as those facilitating reform.

There have been three general trends in the development of health manpower in New York City. Structural pluralism in health training has been somewhat diminished by the increasing leadership of the City University of New York (CUNY). At the lower occupational levels there has been some increased emphasis on training rather than on a direct lateral job entry. However, the effort to ease internal occupational mobility has been counteracted by the efforts of the professional organizations and associations to increase licensing requirements which impede mobility and expansion.

There are five identifiable forces which are working to change or perpetuate arrangements for training allied health manpower. First is the desire of existing professional organizations to maintain and even to raise entrance requirements. There are many associations in the health professions each of which represents a separate field. Physical therapists, occupational therapists, dietitians, social workers, medical technologists, X-ray technicians, and nurses—all have separate organizations to promote their interests. Each seeks to ensure its members a maximum amount of prestige and earning power, both of which are affected by the training required to enter the profession.

A second force shaping the nature of manpower training has been the rapid expansion of programs of the CUNY and the growth of community colleges as training institutions for various fields. From the fall of 1961 to the fall of 1967 the full-time undergraduate population rose from 33,055 to 46,207 at the senior colleges and from 2,293 to 15,617 at the community colleges.[1] As part of this growth the CUNY has instituted new health-related programs and expanded existing ones.

Another factor has been the introduction of federal programs to support the training of allied health manpower. Since 1960 Congress has passed several pieces of legislation aimed at increasing the supply of health and hospital manpower. The most important of these has been the Manpower Development and Training Act (MDTA); others include the Allied Health Professions Training Act, the Nurse Training Act, and the Economic Opportunity Act. Money has been provided to local organizations to train health workers under each of these programs.

A fourth element influencing health training is the recent unionization of large numbers of hospital workers. Since 1965 District Council No. 37 of the American Federation of State, County, and Municipal Employees has represented over 10,000 employees in

the New York City municipal hospitals. In the voluntary and proprietary hospitals, Local 1199 has been conducting a vigorous organizing campaign for several years and now represents employees
in about forty hospitals and nursing homes. While the union's first
priority was to raise hospital workers' wages above their previously
low levels, it has also been concerned with improving training
opportunities for its members.

A final factor has been the increased influence of and concern for
the Negro and Puerto Rican segments of the city's population. One
strategy for improving the status of these citizens has been to provide jobs and opportunities for advancement in existing low-level
occupations. Health services, where many blacks and Puerto Ricans
are already employed, is viewed as an expanding industry where
new jobs will become available.

AN INSTITUTIONAL SHIFT

These five elements have combined in different ways to produce
some broad changes in the nature of training. There has been a
shift from hospitals to educational institutions as the responsible
training organization. Nursing is one field in which this shift is
clearly taking place. As the figures in Table 2.1 indicate, the
number of programs and students enrolled in associate degree or
community college courses has risen rapidly while hospital or

TABLE 2.1

Programs Leading to the Registered Nurse Degree in New York City

	1959			1967			*Percent of Change in En- rollment*
		Enrollment			*Enrollment*		
	Num- ber	*Num- ber*	*Per- cent*	*Num- ber*	*Num- ber*	*Per- cent*	
Diploma schools	30	4,639	79	25	3,876	58	−16
Associate programs	2	198	4	7	1,302	20	+558
Baccalaureate and higher degrees	5	969	17	9	1,464	22	+51
Total	37	5,806	100	41	6,642	100	+14

Source: National League for Nursing, *State Approved Schools of Nursing—RN*,
annual issues.

diploma school programs have decreased in number and enrollment. These figures do not reveal the full strength of the trend. In 1969 the Bellevue School of Nursing graduated its last class; its facilities will henceforth be used by Hunter College to expand its bachelor program. Mount Sinai Hospital has begun phasing out its diploma school and in the future will train nurses in a baccalaureate program administered by City College. These are two of the largest hospital nursing schools in the city.

The forces outlined earlier help explain this change. The American Nurses' Association (ANA) has sought to elevate the professional standing of the occupation by urging that all nurses acquire either an associate or a bachelor's degree. The New York chapter of the ANA has taken the position that no new hospital schools should be opened after 1967 and that existing hospital programs should be transferred to institutions of higher learning by 1972. As the examples of Mount Sinai and Bellevue illustrate, the expanding CUNY has been a willing partner in implementing the ANA's policy. In addition to assuming responsibility for the hospital schools, the CUNY has also expanded associate programs. Table 2.2 shows

TABLE 2.2

Enrollment in CUNY Nursing Programs

College	1959	1967	1972
Hunter	166	473	1,200
Queens	82	126	385
Brooklyn	116		330
City			320
Bronx Community		526	800
Manhattan Community		87	250
Kingsborough Community		145	440
Queensborough Community		150	300
Staten Island Community		130	460
New York City Community		138	420
Community Colleges #7-10			560
Total	364	1,775	5,465

Sources: For 1959 and 1967, the annual issues of the National League for Nursing, *State Approved Schools of Nursing—RN;* for 1972, the Board of Higher Education, *Master Plan of the Board of Higher Education for the City University of New York, 1968,* p. 49.

the CUNY's past and projected enrollment in nursing education. While the university's planners may overestimate the growth of some programs, their total estimate is probably within range. Mount Sinai's School of Nursing had more than 300 students in 1967; City College will certainly have that many. Before Hunter and Bellevue were united, the hospital had a nursing student body of over 650 and the college about 300, so a future enrollment of over 1,000 should be possible. The community colleges have demonstrated a capacity to grow rapidly.

While serving the interests of the ANA and the CUNY this increase in nursing education opportunities also has increased training opportunities for minorities. The growth of associate programs has meant that training time is reduced to two years from the three normally required at a diploma school. This can be an important consideration for those who feel the financial pressure of forgoing employment. Second, hospital schools usually charge tuition while education at the CUNY is tuition-free. This fact may be of limited significance because many hospital school students receive scholarships or loans. However, we can still conclude that the change makes job-required credentials available in a shorter time at an equal or lower cost.

Another point arises from the changing institutional responsibility for training. When training is provided at hospitals, the costs are met by the services provided by the students, tuition fees, and general hospital revenues. In general, tuition fees and the value of student services have not equaled educational costs and hospital schools have operated at a deficit. A study of four diploma schools in the southern New York region revealed that the uncompensated cost to the hospital of graduating one student ranged from $4,353 to $7,065.[2] When nurses are trained at colleges the hospital deficit is eliminated and nursing education is largely financed from tax dollars.

The increased importance of educational institutions in the training of allied health personnel has not been limited to the field of nursing. In recent years occupations for which training was previously acquired at hospitals in an on-the-job or apprenticeship fashion are now represented in programs at community colleges. Programs for medical laboratory technicians and X-ray technicians have been introduced at more than one college and new programs will soon be available in inhalation therapy, medical records, and surgical technology. The Board of Higher Education has also established an Institute of Health Sciences at Hunter College affiliated with the Mount Sinai School of Medicine which will offer baccalaureate training in physical therapy, dietetics, and medical records. The same factors influencing nursing education are at work in these fields: the desire of these organizations to attain the status associated with occupations which require a college degree, short-run economies for hospitals, an expanding university system, and a public commitment to meet the employment needs of the Negro and Puerto Rican communities. The interaction between these last two forces is apparent in the fact that the newly created Eugenio Maria de Hostos Community College, which is to have a concentration of health-related curricula, will be located adjacent to the planned new Lincoln Hospital at 149th Street and Park Avenue in the south Bronx, one of the city's major poverty areas.[3] In addition, former Hunter College President Cross proposed that the building to house the Institute of Health Sciences be constructed in Harlem.[4]

It should be pointed out that savings to hospitals from the shifting of training responsibilities to the colleges are limited; they are short-run economies. Over time, reliance on college training is likely to bestow additional status upon hospital workers and thus raise the wage levels which they can command. Moreover, hospitals have relied on their own programs as a ready supply of labor. In nursing, about three-quarters of the graduates in New York City still come from diploma schools. The rapid phasing out of these facilities would drastically cut the supply of nurses. Thus while the trend is likely to continue, the ANA's target date of 1972 for eliminating hospital schools is unrealistic.

AN INTEREST IN UPGRADING

A second direction of recent change is increased reliance on upgrading as a source of skilled manpower. This means that employers do not rely exclusively upon new graduates without prior work experience as the source of manpower. The new approach recognizes that experience at entry may be related to higher-level job requirements. It leads to the creation of career ladders which have not previously existed in the health field. Nurse's aides can be trained to become Licensed Practical Nurses (LPNs) and eventually Registered Nurses (RNs); lab assistants can be trained to qualify as lab technicians and possibly medical technologists. Similar progressions can be designed in other areas.

Evidence of this trend is found in several places. In the municipal hospitals a program was begun in 1967 which grants nurse's aides time to attend a training program designed by the Board of Education to qualify them as LPNs.[5] Plans are now being made to offer a program to employed LPNs which will enable them to become RNs.[6] In addition, over 1,000 aides have been trained for newly created specialized positions such as obstetrical technician and surgical technician. In the voluntary sector a recent collective bargaining agreement has created a training fund of 1 percent of payroll costs which will be jointly administered by union and hospital officials to provide payments to employees who wish to train for higher-level positions. In 1964 the Helene Fuld School of Nursing was established at the Hospital for Joint Diseases with admission limited to LPNs who want to prepare for the RN exam. At the Albert Einstein College of Medicine a group has been working to develop a training program for Lincoln Hospital based on the principle of career ladders.[7] It is intended that the Eugenio Maria de Hostos Community College will offer special programs designed to permit employed workers to qualify for higher-level jobs.

These plans and initial steps are the result of some of the forces listed earlier, perhaps the most important of which is the unionization of hospital workers. Officials of the American Federation of State, County, and Municipal Employees believe that it was their promise to provide advancement opportunities which enabled them to defeat a Teamsters' local in a hotly contested election for representation. The union formulated plans for the training programs, which were initially established on a demonstration basis but which may become part of collective bargaining agreements. The training fund introduced into a voluntary hospital contract, as described above, was negotiated by Local 1199, which is aggressively organizing lower-echelon workers in the voluntary sector.

Upgrading also represents a conscious effort to provide minorities with meaningful job opportunities. As Table 2.3 indicates, over 80 percent of entering employees at municipal hospitals are either Negro or Puerto Rican. Similar proportions probably exist in most voluntary hospitals. Measures designed to advance the skills of this group produce more RNs and technicians; moreover, they are directed toward raising the income and social status of Negroes and Puerto Ricans. This is evident in the close identification of

TABLE 2.3

*Estimated Ethnic Distribution of Full-Time Workers
in Selected Municipal Hospital Jobs*

	Number Employed	Percent Negro or Puerto Rican
Nurse's aides	8,039	88
Practical nurses	2,731	90
Dietary aides	2,588	84
Housekeeping aides	2,292	80
All entry-job titles	20,071	82

Source: An ethnic census of municipal hospital employees reported in Eleanor Gilpatrick and Paul Corliss, *The Occupational Structure of New York City Municipal Hospitals* (New York: Research Foundation, City University of New York, 1969).

the unions with the civil rights movement. The racial implications of a hospital's policy toward its employees are as evident in New York City as they are in Charleston, South Carolina. However, unlike the hospitals in Charleston, New York's hospitals have dealt with this fact in a more conciliatory fashion. The desire to avoid the racial confrontation which might have resulted from a strike by Local 1199 was an important consideration in the gains the union obtained during its negotiations in 1968 with the League of Voluntary Hospitals, a collective bargaining organization for seventeen hospitals in New York City.

Federal funds have been an important factor in upgrading allied health workers. Although the bulk of federal assistance has not been used for this purpose, the availability of some funds has made it possible for those agencies seeking to provide advancement opportunities to begin to implement their plans. It was only after a federal grant was obtained that the Hospitals Department established its program to train aides to become LPNs. It was an MDTA grant that paid the training expenses to promote aides to the special technical positions. Money for these purposes was simply not available from the tight municipal budget and it was the federal grants which made the innovations possible.

Grants awarded by the Office of Economic Opportunity (OEO) for the creation of neighborhood health centers have frequently included funds for training. These centers have recruited local residents and trained them as family health workers. This is a new job classification predicated on the employee's familiarity with the health needs of the population to be served. Opportunities for such staff to advance are frequently provided through formal programs at neighboring hospitals and educational institutions. These innovative manpower training programs can help to attract new types of personnel into the health field.

These facts should not lead to the conclusion that federal funds have always been used to promote change. Restrictions placed on MDTA on-the-job training grants which limit them to training for nonlicensed or noncertified positions have made the program a training ground for dead-end jobs. As the figures in Table 2.4 indicate, a large part of the training supported by MDTA has been devoted to basic jobs in the housekeeping, food service, and nursing departments, which offer little financial reward or future advancement. In some cases special training programs have been created for jobs which are hardly classifiable as health occupations. For example, funds were used to train about 700 porters and maids, nearly 100 guards and handymen, and about 50 laundry workers. In the majority of cases, MDTA has been a subsidy to hospitals to continue their on-the-job training for entering personnel. It changes the financing, but not the nature, of training for these varied occupations.

While upgrading both generates a supply of skilled manpower

TABLE 2.4

Authorized MDTA On-the-Job Training Positions
January, 1967, to June, 1968

Nursing Department
Nurse's aide	883
Senior nurse's aide	194
Orderly and senior orderly	238
Surgical technician	319
Obstetrical technician	125
Ambulance attendant	341
Ambulatory care aide	65
Other	43
	2,208

Food Service
Dietary aide	348
Senior dietary aide	320
Tray line worker	275
Other kitchen workers	97
	1,040

Housekeeping
Maid and porter	680
Head porter	35
	715

Inhalation Therapy	195

General Services
Communication aide	75
Security guard	44
Utility man and others	59
	178

Clerical
Ward clerk	84
Other clerical	16
	100

Medical Records	52
Laundry Department	48
Medical Laboratory	13
Others	256
Total	4,805

Source: Data supplied by the Social Development Corporation, a prime contractor to the Department of Labor. Figures cover training in New York City only.

and provides jobs for minorities, the two do not always form an ideal package. The goal of meeting manpower shortages has not always received emphasis equal to that of creating jobs. Consequently many people have been trained for new and traditional entry positions, but little effort has been made to follow up with training for advancement to levels requiring more skill. However, it is at the higher levels that more acute shortages exist. For example, in the municipal hospitals the vacancy rate for nurse's aides is only 3 percent and staffing is considered adequate, while the staff nurse (RN) vacancy rate is 27 percent and is considered to be at a chronically critical level.[8] A program to train more aides will do little to relieve staffing problems unless it is accompanied by a program for advancement. Merely "creating jobs" with no regard to the kinds of jobs created does not solve manpower problems. Nor does it always benefit employees. For example, local residents trained for newly established entry positions at an OEO health center have found they cannot readily find employment elsewhere and some have sought training at traditional nursing schools in order to qualify for other jobs. If "new career" programs are to provide employees with meaningful opportunities and to help employers solve staffing problems, they must be related to traditional methods of credentialing.

NEW ENTRANCE STANDARDS

At the same time that efforts have been undertaken to upgrade skills, entrance requirements for professions have been escalated. The two lines of action are strikingly contradictory. The drive to maximize entrance requirements is rooted in the professional organizations. The ANA's call for college preparation for all nurses represents more than a minor institutional shift. Part of its plan is to eliminate existing LPN programs. Under this plan, one could be a nurse with a minimum of just two years of college. This change is not likely to be implemented rapidly because hospital schools still supply many nurses and the LPNs are a large and organized group. However, there are other areas where opposition to raising entrance requirements has not existed or has not been effective.

Professional organizations of pharmacists were successful in raising entrance requirements so that a pharmacy education now consists of a total of five years of college. This standard was set in the early 1960s when the course of study was lengthened from four years. It is interesting to note that this change was implemented while enrollment in pharmacy schools was declining. From 1960 to 1967 enrollment in the four pharmacy schools in New York City declined by almost 40 percent (Table 2.5). It is un-

TABLE 2.5

Enrollment in Pharmacy Programs in New York City

	1960–61	1967–68
Columbia University		
Senior year	92	47
Total	302	176
Fordham University		
Senior year	95	37
Total	283	138
St. John's University		
Senior year	69	46
Total	257	198
Long Island University–Brooklyn		
Senior year	116	89
Total	392	270
Total, four schools		
Senior year	372	219
Total	1,234	782

Source: Figures reported annually in the *American Journal of Pharmaceutical Education*. "Total" refers to the last three years of the collegiate program.

doubtedly true that other factors, including competition for students from other scientific disciplines and an image of the pharmacist as a neighborhood businessman, help explain this decline. Nonetheless the fact that entrance requirements were raised in the face of declining enrollment and increasing needs is an indication of the strength of professional organizations.

Another example of escalating entrance requirements can be found in the training of X-ray technicians.[9] In 1964 the New York State legislature enacted a law requiring that all X-ray technicians be licensed. The adoption of the licensure law and its more stringent standards can be attributed to an alliance between the Society of X-Ray Technicians and the New York State Department of Health. The society was interested in enforcing higher standards in order to upgrade the profession. Part of the Health Department's mission was to protect the public from dangers of excessive radiation and it was felt this could best be accomplished by ensuring that the operators of X-ray equipment were properly trained. Together the two organizations were able to convince the legislature to change the existing requirements.

This change affected the locus of training. As a result of the state licensure law and a somewhat similar New York City ordinance concerning medical laboratory technicians, relevant training programs of private or commercial schools have been curtailed. Prior to enactment of the state law there were four commercial schools offering X-ray technician training with a student capacity described by the State Health Department as "unknown but large." These schools were disqualified for training by the statute because they could not offer the required clinical experience. Private schools in New York City no longer train any X-ray technicians. According to a city regulation, medical laboratory technicians are licensed after they complete an approved two-year course or pass an examination. Therefore, individuals who go to a community college automatically get a license while those who study at a private school must pass the exam. This fact, added to differences in tuition between community colleges and private schools, places the latter at a disadvantage in recruiting students. By 1967 there were about 300 students at four community college programs for laboratory technicians. Since both types of institution draw students primarily from recent high school graduates, the private schools have suffered as the community colleges have grown.

RESISTANCE TO CHANGE

Several aspects of the structure of training have prevented the expansion of training. The fact that MDTA has often provided financial support for existing patterns of on-the-job training rather than for new programs has already been noted. The city's vocational high schools have made similarly meager contributions. In the 1960s virtually no change took place in the size or scope of vocational high school training for health-related occupations. Figures provided by the Board of Education show that enrollment in health-related programs at New York City vocational high schools was 3,066 in 1961 and 2,801 in 1967. In both years this represents about 7 percent of all vocational high school students.

As mentioned earlier, the dominant trend has been that occupational organizations have pressed for college-based training. This has left the high schools with few opportunities for expansion. At present most high school students interested in health-related careers are enrolled in programs which qualify them for entry-level hospital jobs. The programs have not grown because graduates must still undergo the same training as other newly employed aides; they are not eligible for any jobs for which other high school graduates are not qualified. In addition, the city's black population has been negative toward the Board of Education and those sympathetic to their aspirations are not likely to seek expansion of institutions under the Board's control. Therefore it has been the community colleges which have offered continuing education programs and supplied staff for training in municipal hospitals. It is also anticipated that a branch of the CUNY will take over from the Board of Education the LPN training program for employed aides.

One exception to the rule of minimal change in the city's high schools is the training of practical nurses. In this case graduates are qualified for positions for which others are not and the training produces valuable credentials. From 1960 to 1967 additional programs for LPNs were provided at both vocational and academic high schools and during these years total enrollment in these programs increased from 405 to 610.[10]

The development of training facilities may be impeded by professional rivalries. For over a decade the New York State Optometric Association, and particularly the staff of the Optometric Center of New York City, sought to establish an optometry school in the state.[11] The need for such a school appears to exist. Over 200 students from New York attend schools in other parts of the country and almost one-third of the students at schools in Pennsylvania and Massachusetts are New York residents. Leaders of the optometrists' group presented their argument to the Board of Regents and to officials of both the State and City University systems. In each instance failure to act was attributed to resistance from ophthalmologists. The ophthalmologists and the optometrists are engaged in continuing battle. Optometrists operate as independent practitioners who examine eyes, prescribe glasses, and treat some disorders by recommending visual exercises. Opthalmologists perform the same functions but are also qualified to treat a wider range of diseases, prescribe drugs, and perform surgery. They argue that optometrists are not trained as thoroughly and should practice only under an ophthalmologist's supervision. The optometrists counter that they are adequately prepared to perform the functions which they are legally permitted to do. They believe that ophthalmologists oppose their role as independent practitioners for economic reasons. A large part of many ophthalmologists' practice consists of eye examinations and refractions, tasks for which optometrists compete with them. The continuing battle between the two professions produced a stalemate until 1970 when the state created a school under the trusteeship of the Optometric Center. However, it is still not possible to locate the school at any existing university or medical school campus and the absence of suitable facilities will make it difficult to meet the commitment to admit the first class in 1971.

In addition to fighting the establishment of training facilities for competing occupational groups, entrenched professional organizations have been able to prevent changes in state licensing requirements. With the exception of the new law concerning X-ray technicians, little change has taken place. This is so primarily because the licensing bodies are isolated from the new pressures for change. In almost all fields, requirements are set by a Board of Examiners. Its members are appointed by the Board of Regents, which is elected by the state legislature. It is common practice, in some cases because of statutory provisions and in others because of tradition and political influence, for the Board of Examiners in each field to be dominated by members of the profession and usually by leaders of the professional organization. Therefore, decisions on licensing requirements have reflected existing professional opinion and are kept immune from the influence of other forces. Recently Local 1199 has begun to advocate changes in the composition of some Boards of Examiners and it is possible that in the future there will be efforts to include more interest groups on these bodies.

The existing system of training allied health manpower has demonstrated an ability to adjust to the industry's growing needs. The continuing expansion of the city's educational institutions and an increased reliance on upgrading have significantly enlarged the number of individuals trained. In occupations which have not increased, severe problems have been avoided because of New York's ability to attract individuals trained elsewhere. For example, in the 1960s additions to New York's optometrists were supplied entirely by other states. In 1967 New York State issued 7,835 new licenses to registered nurses; over 3,000 of these went to individuals previously licensed in another state or a foreign country.[12] New York was surpassed only by California in its ability to attract trained nurses.

The diverse cluster of activity known as the training of allied health manpower has experienced both stasis and change. In the past decade a shift in training from hospital to college has begun, upgrading has been identified as a potential source of skilled manpower, and entrance requirements for some occupations have been raised and formalized. In the midst of these changes there exist islands of inflexibility. The state remains without an active optometry school, vocational high schools continue their minor role in supplying manpower, and most licensing requirements are still immune to change. Each instance of change or inflexibility results primarily from the impact of one or more of these forces—the control of professional organizations over entrance standards, the rapid expansion of the City University's educational complex, the availability of federal assistance, the unionization of hospital workers, and a commitment to expand employment opportunities for the city's Negro and Puerto Rican population.

3

CAPITAL FUNDING

THE QUANTITY and the quality of health services provided to the people of New York City are partly a function of the amount, the distribution, and the state of repair of its health plant and equipment. The cost of providing those services is also affected by plant and equipment—their age and design, the size of the individual units, and spatial dispersion. Health services are produced by human and physical resources; it is physical resources with which we are concerned here.

Specifically, we wish to know the sources and uses of capital funds flowing into the health facilities in New York City. Further, we are concerned with the forces which influence the amounts of capital funds and their allocation among alternative (and often competing) facilities. Ultimately, we want to determine whether the capital flows are adequate both in amount and in distribution to provide, together with other input factors, an optimum level of health care for the people of the metropolis at or near minimum cost levels. We shall attempt here only to bring out some of the highlights.

A good indication of the state of our knowledge in these matters is the state of the basic data: they do not exist in the form needed to answer the questions just posed. There is no central agency, private or public, in New York City which now can provide internally consistent, comprehensive data on capital investment in health plant and equipment. This is due, in large part, to the pluralistic nature of the control systems in health—that is, to the combination of federal, state, municipal, voluntary (nonprofit), and proprietary institutions that constitute our health facilities (see chapter 1). When we add to this the lack of uniform accounting and reporting procedures among these institutions, we can begin to appreciate the dimensions of the task.

It is only within the last several years, for example, that hospitals began to submit comprehensive data on a "Uniform Statistical Report for Hospitals" to the Health and Hospital Planning Council of Southern New York, although the United Hospital Fund has been getting some data of this type from the voluntary hospitals. Several of the questions in this report pertain to construction activity but these have not yet been summarized or analyzed. It is also possible to purchase from the F. W. Dodge Corporation a special tabulation of the value of construction contracts let by New York City hospitals, but this does not include all health facilities and is available only for recent years. Finally, we must distinguish between contracts let and actual brick and mortar put in place, or, as in the municipal budget, between authorized and actual expenditures. This task of data collection is laborious; it has not been done but it is a first-priority job that needs to be done on a continuing basis if we are to have meaningful analyses of capital flows into New York City's health system.

A second priority task, almost equally important, is the maintenance of a "perpetual inventory" of the age distribution of facilities and of the extent of functional obsolescence. Determination of the latter is difficult since it depends on the criteria used to determine functional obsolescence and there may be valid professional disagreement on this point. Profit-seeking firms are under market pressures which force them to maintain such inventories, but since health facilities are primarily governed by criteria of social utility, calculations such as return on investment, marginal efficiency of capital, payback periods, and competitive evaluations are seldom if ever made.

One other general note concerning investment in plant and equipment. The economist distinguishes gross from net investment; that is, only when annual gross investment exceeds annual depreciation does he say that positive net capital formation has occurred. In the health field, however, an increase in the number of beds is a measure conventionally used to indicate an increase in (gross) investment. But there are many pitfalls in this practice. For instance, an actual decrease in the number of beds may result from an increase in investment, as when a ward facility is converted to semiprivate or private accommodations. Conversely, an increase in bed complement may result from a change in function of a department (say, from maternity to general care) without significant, if any, additions to plant and equipment. Moreover, huge investment in the modernization of health facilities may be made without a change in the number of beds; again, a new research facility may be constructed which contains no beds. In addition, since an increasing amount of health services is rendered on an outpatient or ambulatory basis, the bed measure loses even more of its strength as an index of the use of health plant and equipment. It appears, then, that we ought to move toward a net capital formation concept of investment in the health field, although this does not mean that we should abandon the bed measure altogether—it still is essential for many analytical purposes.

THE STATE OF THE HOSPITAL PLANT

IN NEW YORK CITY

The most recent study of the physical state of general care hospitals in New York City (excluding nursing homes, chronic disease and mental hospitals, clinics, etc.) offers evidence that depreciation and functional obsolescence have proceeded at faster rates than capital funds have been accumulated.[1] The authors of that report (Friedman and Colman) state that, in 1965, it would have required $700 million to effect needed replacements and renovations, without providing new or expanded hospital services or acquiring new sites or ancillary services (parking space, etc.). Among the criteria employed to determine needs for replacement and repair were the extent of overcrowding; the degree to which hospitals were protected against fire, explosive hazards, and infection; the presence of specialized facilities for ambulant or wheelchair patients; the presence of emergency electrical power supply; physical deterioration; and the presence of minimal amenities to ensure patient privacy. The senior author of the report recently stated that the basic situation had worsened in the interim. With construction costs having increased by at least 30 percent over the intervening four years, the replacement cost in 1969 would surely have exceeded $1 billion—for general care hospitals alone.

Highly significant was the number of hospitals that were judged by the authors to be beyond repair and which, therefore, warranted complete replacement—33 percent of all the voluntary hospitals (26 out of 78); 52 percent of all municipal hospitals (9 out of 17); and 34 percent of the proprietaries (12 out of 35). The municipal figure is particularly surprising since during the postwar years 1945–56 more capital funds flowed into the municipal hospitals than into the voluntary sector.[2]

To sum up, New York City has some of the best and most modern general care hospitals in the country, if not in the world (Columbia-Presbyterian Medical Center, Mount Sinai, New York Hospital–Cornell, New York University–Bellevue, etc.), but it also has some of the worst—and the distribution is skewed uncomfortably toward the poor end of the spectrum.

So much for the general dimensions of the problem; we turn now to some of the specifics of the major sources of capital flows into New York City's health plant.

CAPITAL FUNDS FLOW FROM
THE CITY BUDGET

The intricate, tortuous, and time-consuming trail that leads from departmental requests to actual construction in New York City is well known. Professor Yavitz and others of my colleagues present some case studies relating to this issue elsewhere in this volume.

At this point some benchmark data for purposes of perspective are relevant. Table 3.1 shows capital funds allocated to expenditures and actual expenditures for health facilities for selected years from 1950–51 to 1967–68. These data are from the so-called Capital Improvement accounts in the City Budget and comprise all of the spending or authorizations to spend by all departments for health construction purposes—primarily the Department of Hospitals, Health, and Public Works. It should be emphasized here that these figures are capital funds and not expense or operating funds, which

TABLE 3.1

New York City Capital Budget Authorizations Allocated for Expenditures and Expenditures by Nature of Improvement

	1950–51	1955–56	1960–61	1965–66	1967–68
Authorizations allocated for expenditures					
Health and teaching centers	$ 588,397	$ 309,441	$ 142,840	$ 3,056,650	$ 4,958,892
Hospitals and allied buildings	62,222,817	7,320,583	10,304,154	81,900,928	54,993,930
Total—health and hospitals	62,811,214	7,630,024	10,446,994	84,957,578	59,952,822
Total—all capital improvements	262,378,009	343,894,874	432,702,714	504,049,602	1,022,110,107
Health and hospitals as a percent of total	23.9	2.2	2.4	16.9	5.9
Expenditures					
Health and teaching centers	$ 690,003	$ 1,278,784	$ 498,433	$ 5,970,436	$ 2,778,988
Hospitals and allied buildings	13,047,447	22,241,735	9,206,924	20,137,162	40,549,648
Total—health and hospitals	13,737,450	23,520,519	9,705,357	26,107,598	43,328,636
Total—all capital improvements	202,396,903	315,999,755	315,757,272	465,783,818	487,149,376
Health and hospitals as a percent of total	6.8	7.4	3.1	5.6	8.9

Source: Annual Reports of the Comptroller of the City of New York.

are much larger. In 1968, for instance, the city budgeted about $885 million for the production of personal health care.

The municipality, it should be noted, operates some 18 hospitals and medical centers with a complement of over 17,000 beds, or 25 percent of the total beds in the city, in addition to Health Department clinics, neighborhood health centers, community mental health centers, and the office of the Chief Medical Examiner.

Table 3.1 is interesting from a number of viewpoints. The upper panel represents authorizations to spend—that is, capital projects which have been approved and for which funds have been put aside to be spent in the future. The lower panel shows actual expenditures at the time of disbursement. The reason that an "expenditure" may exceed an authorization is that expenditures reflect outlays for projects and phases of construction initiated in prior years. Total authorizations to spend show large variations in the period covered—a high of approximately $85 million in 1965–66 and a low of $7.6 million in 1955–56. As a percentage of all capital improvements, the variations are also great—a high of 23.9 percent in 1950–51 and a low of 2.2 percent in 1955–56. The variations in actual expenditures are, by comparison, quite small—a range of 3.1 to 8.9 percent. This suggests that the city is able to arrange for payments of a large total project cost over a series of years whereas large portions of the total cost of a project appear as an authorization in the budget of a single year (see Yavitz's comments on the budgetary process).

Nevertheless, capital expenditures for health are not uniquely related to, say, population growth. They are a complex function of the quantity, types, and ages of existing facilities and of the quantity and types and costs of new ones. Moreover, there is always competition for city capital funds from schools, police and sanitation services, housing, highways, and the like.

Many of the recent investigations of the city's health affairs, including the Mayor's Task Force on Medical Economics and the report on *Comprehensive Community Health Services for New York City* (Piel Report), have recommended a new corporate authority for the municipal hospital system which would be unencumbered by current constraints. Such a body would be able to cut red tape and would be free of city debt limits; it could raise funds by the sale of bonds and notes in the capital markets when the need arose rather than when funds happen to be available. Long-range planning would thereby become feasible. A bill authorizing such a body was passed by the state legislature and was signed into law by the governor. On July 1, 1970, the New York City Department of Hospitals was replaced by the New York City Health and Hospitals Corporation, which will be responsible for the operation of the municipal hospital system. The Health Services Administrator will be a member of the board of directors and new relationships will have to be forged with the comprehensive health-planning agency to be appointed under Public Law 89-749 as well as with the agency presently administering the state Metcalf-McClosky and Folsom laws (see below), namely, the Health and Hospital Planning Council of Southern New York, Inc. Once these knotty problems are disentangled, New York City may be on the road to achieving a more rational and systematic program of capital flows into its health facilities.

Long-range investment programs for health services were also brought closer to realization by the inclusion in Medicare and Medicaid reimbursement formulas of allowances for depreciation and for debt servicing charges. Since all types of facilities, public and private, that provide services under these programs will receive such funds, the need for emergency fund raising may diminish.

We can foresee, then, some resolution of the bureaucratic difficulties and some improvement resulting from placing capital financing on a more current basis via reimbursement. On the other hand, the bond-issuing capacity of the new Health and Hospitals Corporation is more apparent than real. Under current legislation the city retains ownership of the hospital plant but will not pledge its credit to back up the Corporation's bonds. Without one or the other, the Corporation cannot raise funds. It is questionable, therefore, whether the city can establish an adequate financial base for its ambitious programs of renovation and replacement of existing hospitals and for the initiation and carrying through of programs for ambulatory patients, such as the neighborhood family care centers and community mental health centers. The capital funds required for these programs are sizable. It is estimated that the "accelerated renovation" of sixteen hospitals will cost $65 million and that the ambulatory care facilities program will involve a capital investment of $100 million.[3] Unless large and continuing amounts of state and federal aid are made available, the city will continue to be in the grip of a "scissors crisis," that is, rapidly rising costs and utilization on the one hand and a tight budget on the other.

CAPITAL FUNDS FROM FEDERAL SOURCES

The federal government operates relatively few hospitals in the New York City area. There are three Veterans Administration hospitals, a Public Health Service hospital, and a Naval health facility. Together these have about 5,000 beds, while all other hospital beds in the city total approximately 64,000. But the federal role extends beyond the institutions under federal control, especially since the passage of the Hill-Burton legislation of 1946 and the important amendments thereto. New York City has not been an important beneficiary of Hill-Burton funds ($50 million over a fifteen-year period) in part because the original legislation aimed at rectifying rural hospital deficiencies first and in part because New York State's participation was limited by the per capita income requirements of the aid formula. Hill-Burton's effect on city construction was therefore more qualitative than quantitative. In the first place, the act mandated the establishment of state plans for hospital dispersion and high construction standards. Secondly, capital funds were allocated to New York City so as to help remedy imbalances in bed totals among the five boroughs. Of the 3,000 or so general care beds whose construction was aided by Hill-Burton funds through 1963, 42 percent were in Queens, 6 percent in Richmond, 19 percent in the Bronx, 25 percent in Kings (Brooklyn), and 8 percent in Manhattan. Thirdly, Hill-Burton funds promoted the establishment of special types of beds which were in short supply, for example, premature infant units, beds for mental patients, and beds for chronic invalids.

The Nixon Administration proposed that construction and modernization grants under Hill-Burton funds be replaced by a $500 million annual loan (guarantee) program, with emphasis shifting away from hospitals toward outpatient clinics, neighborhood health centers, nursing homes, and other nonhospital health facilities. The intent was to offer less expensive alternatives to inpatient care as well as to promote preventive care. This type of shift would operate to the benefit of New York City, which is committed to the development of ambulatory care programs. However, compromise legislation enacted by Congress in 1970, over presidential veto, has extended through 1973 the traditional construction grant program, supplemented by a substantial mortgage loan guarantee authorization and interest subsidy. Although still a minor competitor for funds, ambulatory facilities are receiving a substantially increased share and there has been some liberalization in the law to include nonhospital-connected diagnostic and therapeutic facilities.

In addition to the Hill-Burton legislation, the last few years have witnessed a proliferation of new federal programs designed to channel capital funds into health facilities. These include, among others, the Health Professions Educational Assistance Act of 1963, the Economic Opportunity Act of 1963, the Community Mental Health Center Construction Act of 1963, the Mental Retardation Facilities Construction Act of 1963, and the programs of the Department of Housing and Urban Development such as Model Cities. Most of this legislation is designed to assist public and nonprofit institutions, but loans are available to proprietary health facilities through the Small Business Administration as well as under the National Housing Act.

Table 3.2 presents a summary of capital funds flowing into New York State and New York City under the various grant programs of the United States Public Health Service over the six-year period 1961-66. We note, first, that New York City, with approximately 4 percent of the nation's population, received 2.5 percent of the funds under these programs. Secondly, the absolute amounts were not large. Given the relatively high construction costs in the city, it is not possible to do much in the way of hospital and medical facilities construction (under Hill-Burton authorization) with an average of $1 million per year (25 beds at $40,000 per bed). With individual programs New York City fared relatively well, receiving,

TABLE 3.2

New York City's Share of Facilities Grants by U.S.
Public Health Service, 1961–1966
(in millions of dollars)

	Total (6 years)	Percent of Total Grants	Percent of Grants by Program
All grant programs			
United States	$1,617.2	100.0	100.0
New York State	101.6	6.3	6.3
New York City	39.7	2.5	2.5
Health research facilities			
United States	273.7	16.9	100.0
New York State	42.0	2.6	15.3
New York City	24.3	1.5	8.9
Health-related teaching facilities			
United States	172.2	10.6	100.0
New York State	2.8	.2	1.6
New York City	1.1	.1	.6
Hospital and medical facilities construction			
United States	1,074.9	66.5	100.0
New York State	47.0	2.9	4.4
New York City	6.1	.4	.6
Mental retardation research facilities			
United States	54.8	3.4	100.0
New York State	6.9	.4	12.6
New York City	6.2	.4	11.3
Community mental health centers			
United States	41.8	2.6	100.0
New York State	2.9	.2	6.9
New York City	2.0	.1	4.8

Source: Adapted from Charlotte Muller, "Program Elements of Federal Laws on Financing of Health Facilities" (Center for Social Research, City University of New York, October 10, 1962), p. 24. Figures may not total because of rounding.

for example, 8.9 percent of the total amount allocated as health research facilities funds and 11.3 percent of all mental retardation research facilities funds.

There is thus no shortage of programs but, as we have noted, the funds allocated (at least from 1961 to 1966) could not provide adequate implementation of the programs. Moreover, the federal share of a project is usually limited either by the enabling legislation or by administrative rulings to a variable fraction of its total cost. (The federal share of an individual project is limited to one-third in New York State.) Grants usually must be matched and loans must be repaid, although forgiveness loans and moratoria may be easier to obtain from the federal government than from other sources. Finally, many facilities may have been built because the funds acted as a catalyst but little or no provision was made for other input factors such as manpower. It appears that some of the OEO neighborhood health centers in New York City and elsewhere may already be in this position.

Students of governmental economic policy are aware of the problems that can be generated when there are multiple funding sources for a given program. Some of the programs mentioned above deal with states alone, some with states and localities, while still others bypass intermediate political levels and reach directly into the communities. This can and does cause confusion and it makes coordination extremely difficult to achieve. It may be wiser to have fewer, synchronized programs than many uncoordinated ones. The city, in attempting to take advantage of the extent and variety of programs available, may find itself with many starts but few completions.

CAPITAL FLOWS FROM STATE SOURCES

The state government, which has control of some 15,000 beds in New York City, is more directly involved than the federal government in the New York City health picture. The fact that almost all of these beds are in a few relatively large mental hospitals, however, tends to narrow the focus of state responsibility for general inpatient health care.

Nevertheless, the state exercises a profound degree of control over all of New York City's health facilities by virtue of the powers vested in the State Health Department, the State Department of Social Welfare, and the State Hospital Review and Planning Council by both the state constitution and such legislation as the Metcalf-McClosky and Folsom amendments to the state's Public Health and

Social Welfare Laws. These acts stipulate, in general terms, that all applications by hospitals and nursing homes for modernization or new construction must receive prior approval of the State Commissioner of Health. The State Health Department also administers Hill-Burton disbursements in New York. These rather comprehensive state powers are delegated in the case of New York City to the Health and Hospital Planning Council of Southern New York, Inc., a nonprofit agency which has been in existence since 1937. However, recent developments with regard to the designation of the City of New York as the comprehensive health-planning agency for the area under federal law (Public Law 89-749) have introduced complications with respect to the existing legal and administrative structures just outlined.

The basic criterion used by the Planning Council in determining whether application for capital spending by an institution should be approved is whether the action will help move the institution toward the "medical service center" concept, that is, a relatively large facility (minimum of 400 beds) capable of providing a broad spectrum of services on the "progressive patient care" principle—from ambulatory diagnostic services to chronic care and geriatric services. Obviously not every application for the renovation of a floor or for the installation of new equipment meets the criterion, but large-scale ones may. With regard to nursing homes, the Council favors those with hospital affiliations (public or voluntary), but since the majority of these facilities are proprietary in nature, the Council has had few alternatives from which to choose. The four to five years during which the Council has utilized its broad powers are too few to have effected any basic changes in the configuration of New York City's health facilities. Its planning posture is more negative than positive since it cannot initiate projects but can only pass on applications submitted to it. Most of its actions, as can be seen from recent annual reports, concern applications for construction at existing institutions. Some recent exceptions are for construction of new nursing homes and neighborhood family care centers.

Until the passage of a constitutional amendment in November, 1969, the state was precluded from making construction funds available to voluntary institutions. Hence, its extension of capital funds has been in the form of state aid given directly to local governments, long-term low-interest loans for the construction of nursing home facilities under the Nursing Home Companies Law (1966), and state reimbursement to localities of up to one-third the cost of construction of public nursing homes, community mental health centers, and hostels for the mentally retarded.

A new state program of potentially large significance ($700 million in funds have been authorized) enables the State Housing Finance Agency to finance construction of municipal health facilities (broadly defined to include ancillary facilities) on condition that they be built by the State Health and Mental Hygiene Facilities Improvement Corporation. Under this program, capital-starved municipalities like New York City do not have to invest capital but may lease facilities and repay the loan later out of current income derived from operating the facility. The city receives full title after the bonds are paid off. A constitutional amendment approved in the November, 1969, elections extends this program to voluntary hospitals with a bond authorization totaling $350 million.

The first project under the municipal program was begun in September, 1969. Ground was broken for the new North Central Bronx Hospital, a 412-bed, $92,750,000 facility designed also to accommodate in its outpatient clinic up to 800 patients a day, or a quarter of a million annually. Two additional hospitals, Lincoln Medical Center in the Bronx and Greenpoint Medical Center in Brooklyn, are scheduled, as well as four Neighborhood Family Care Centers in Brownsville, lower Washington Heights, and the Longwood and Morrisania sections of the Bronx.

Many of the programs mentioned are too new to have generated data on funds actually expended under them but they have the potential for creating a sizable increase in the flow of capital to New York City health facilities.

INTERNAL AND EXTERNAL FINANCING

BY VOLUNTARY AND PROPRIETARY

HEALTH FACILITIES

In New York City, publicly controlled hospital beds (federal, state, and city) constitute 54 percent of the total bed complement, beds under voluntary auspices amount to about 39 percent, and those in proprietary institutions account for some 7 percent of the total. Although they control a minority of the beds, the voluntary hospitals occupy a strategic role in the health economy of the city. For the most part they are general hospitals; several of them are part of large hospital–medical school complexes; some are teaching hospitals and many engage in extensive medical research. Perhaps it is because of these factors that each institution guards its autonomy closely, with the result that there is little cooperation among them and not a little competition for specialists, programs, and funds. Certainly their capital investment plans are not coordinated. Each hospital makes its own investment decisions based on such considerations as its size, its age, its programs (current and projected), and the availability of funds whether from internal sources (surpluses generated from patient revenues) or from external sources such as philanthropy, long- and short-term borrowing, equity financing, and grants or loans from public sources such as the programs discussed above. As was already noted, reimbursement formulas now include allowances for capital costs so that a greater proportion of capital funds will henceforth be derived from current operating income. Current Blue Cross practice permits reimbursement for depreciation and rental expense up to 6 percent of total operating expense.

To determine whether current investment levels are adequate to (at least) maintain the integrity of existing plant and equipment, we shall use the procedure mentioned earlier, namely, calculate the extent to which annual gross investment exceeds or falls short of annual depreciation. Let us see how the voluntary hospitals fare on this basis.

In 1963 Klarman used a figure of $25,000 to represent the cost of new hospital construction on a per bed basis.[4] On the assumption that construction costs have risen about 7.5 percent per annum since then, the cost would now (1969) be approximately $36,000. If we then multiply this number by the approximately 27,000 voluntary beds in New York City, we arrive at a figure of $972 million as the current value (replacement cost) of hospital plant. Using the 3 percent annual depreciation factor applied by Rorem,[5] we find that this plant depreciates each year by some $29 million at current prices.

Annual gross investment, henceforth, must exceed this figure in order for positive capital formation to occur. The only internally consistent series of gross investments by voluntary hospitals that is available is that derived by Muller and Worthington from a study of forty of the largest voluntary hospitals. We can infer from their data, shown in Table 3.3, that gross investment must have exceeded depreciation in recent years since the figures, derived from forty hospitals, represent less than the total voluntary bed complement and the number and value of the beds was lower in earlier years. No

TABLE 3.3

Total Gross Investment for Forty Voluntary Hospitals, 1946–1965

Year	Gross Investment	Year	Gross Investment
1946	$ 1,261,379	1956	$ 8,788,423
1947	2,367,903	1957	14,519,396
1948	4,425,011	1958	20,641,059
1949	7,762,421	1959	17,675,633
1950	10,282,013	1960	15,404,627
1951	15,375,865	1961	26,480,726
1952	10,410,972	1962	28,889,981
1953	14,279,434	1963	36,625,322
1954	11,929,146	1964	38,333,310
1955	21,926,987	1965	32,954,581

Source: Charlotte Muller and Paul Worthington, "Factors Entering into Capital Decisions of Hospitals," paper prepared for the Second Conference on the Economics of Health, December 5-7, 1968, at the Johns Hopkins University, p. 34.

precise statement can be made unless separate calculations are performed for each year. However, the 1965 hospital obsolescence study cited earlier leads one to conclude that there was considerable underinvestment (or negative net capital formation) in voluntary hospitals in the past, to wit: "The elimination of major plant deficiencies, excluding those related to staff housing and research, in each of the 58 voluntary hospitals in New York City would require the total replacement of 14 hospitals and some renovation at each of the remaining 44 hospitals. The total cost of accomplishing this is estimated to be $345,300,000."[6]

These calculations, it should be noted, refer to the maintenance of an existing capital stock; they shed no light on such questions as location, function, utilization, and possible duplication of facilities and equipment—questions which are beyond the purview of this chapter.

With regard to the sources of funds, Rorem has estimated that, for voluntary hospitals on a national basis, approximately 22 percent of capital funds are derived from governmental sources, about 41 percent from philanthropy, and about 37 percent from borrowing, reserves, and miscellaneous sources.[7]

Unfortunately, we do not have the corresponding percentages for New York City but some of the evidence presented above permits certain inferences. We have seen that relatively little federal money entered the New York City hospital economy and no state or city funds were available to voluntary hospitals for capital purposes (exclusive of attached nursing homes which are eligible for low-cost loans). We surmise, therefore, that no more than 5 or 10 percent of the capital funds expended by voluntary hospitals came from governmental sources directly; the overwhelming amounts were derived from philanthropy, borrowing, reserves, endowment funds, and current surpluses. One economist estimated that, in 1960, 94 percent of the book value of the plant assets of 42 voluntary hospitals in New York City was hospital-owned and 6 percent was borrowed; in 1965, 91 percent of the equity was hospital-owned and 9 percent borrowed.[8] In the future, the percentage of capital funds derived from hospital reserves and from borrowing should increase, since depreciation allowances and interest on borrowed capital are reimbursable expenses under current formulas.

Proprietary hospitals, nursing homes, and convalescent centers are not eligible for governmental capital funds and must rely on their own internally generated funds, on borrowing, or on equity financing in the capital markets; usually they use a combination of all three.

The factors to which we have alluded, namely, autonomy, competition, *ad hoc* fund raising, and lack of coordination of investment plans among voluntary and proprietary hospitals, have led to the duplication and consequent underutilization of expensive plant and equipment, to a less than optimum geographic distribution of facilities, and to a general impairment of plant.[9] The fact that municipal facilities may be worse in these respects adds to the discomfiture.

CONCLUDING REMARKS

The last part of this chapter summarizes, somewhat more freely than is customary, the material which was given a broad-brush treatment above. Some of the following statements derive rather directly from the material reviewed, while others are implied in the general statements that were made.

1. Without further elaboration here we wish to stress again the need for comprehensive data collection by a central agency on capital outlays for health services.

2. Any analysis of capital policies is neutral with respect to control. Plant and equipment must be maintained and expanded irrespective of whether they are owned by a municipality or by a voluntary or proprietary group. Control enters this analysis only in so far as it promotes or inhibits optimum investment and reinvestment policies. The evidence reviewed indicates that, despite a new facility here and there, all three types of hospitals—municipal, voluntary, and proprietary—have been deficient in this regard.

3. An optimum investment policy may require the closing of obsolete facilities, cost-saving mergers, and the relocation of other facilities in accordance with demographic and epidemiological changes. These steps are difficult to accomplish but can be made easier if the community is convinced that the policy-making agency places the community's interest above any other considerations. If a facility can no longer be used as a general care hospital, perhaps with some additional investment it can be converted to a diagnostic or mental health clinic. All alternatives of this kind must be considered. It is of the utmost importance to have a "health presence"— some type of facility, however small—in every well-defined neighborhood. It should be noted, however, that rehabilitation of older facilities may not cost significantly less than building anew, and to tax-weary residents this can be a potent argument in support of facility closings.

4. Investment policy must be dovetailed with manpower policy. New facilities or additions to older facilities which are inoperative or which may not attract sufficient personnel should be avoided.

5. Investment planning on a long-range, area-wide basis must supplant autonomous decisions. It is incumbent on a health-planning agency to decide: (a) where and when to erect a new plant; (b) under what conditions to keep an old plant going; (c) whether to remodel plants in accordance with changing health needs and technological advances; (d) when to increase the capital plant by the addition of more equipment; (e) how to balance higher labor costs in inefficient facilities with potential costs in new facilities; (f) when to close down.

6. One of the important problems facing health planners is the fact that the pace of technology may make a structure obsolete before it is completed. Therefore more attention needs to be paid to design problems—to the time consumed and to the flexibility of the end product.

7. Since capital policy involves durable equipment as well as plant, planning for the widespread use of computers in health facilities should be accelerated.

When all these factors are considered, money is a necessary but not a sufficient condition for optimum investment policies.

4

MANAGING
CAPITAL PROJECTS

AN OBSERVER at the opening of the new Harlem Hospital concluded his reminiscences with "Well, here it is. Finally! But it sure took a long time to get here." Indeed the emergence of any municipal hospital, or the major capital addition to one, represents the culmination of a long and tortuous path. The folklore of capital projects in New York City is replete with incidents of postponements, delays, changes, and reversals. A brief, and somewhat impressionistic, review of Harlem Hospital's history will highlight many of the incidents and frustrations, and "flesh out" the essentially abstract process known as capital budgeting and construction.

THE LONG WINDING ROAD—
A CASE HISTORY

In September, 1969, when our observer believed that the hospital was completed, his comment was premature. The newly opened main building was, in fact, only one part of the planned complex of the new Harlem Hospital Center. As Tables 4.1 and 4.2 indicate, its origin can be traced back to the capital budget of 1952, which appropriated $110,000 of an estimated total need of $5,310,000 toward the reconstruction of and additions to the then existing hospital buildings. These funds, plus approximately $30,000 added in 1953, were used for the formulation of plans and designs. In 1954 an appropriation of over $6 million was made for actual construction, the estimated total cost of which had by then risen by about one and a half million dollars.

TABLE 4.1
Harlem Hospital Project, Yearly Data

Time Period	Capital Budget Adoptions	Amount of Adoption Initiated	Time Period	Amount Authorized for Expenditure	Actual Expenditure
1/1/52–12/31/52	$ 110,000	$ 110,000	7/1/52–6/30/53	$ 140,000	$ 27,083
1/1/53–12/31/53	45,000	30,000	7/1/53–6/30/54		43,007
1/1/54–12/31/54	6,060,000		7/1/54–6/30/55	6,692,000	78,834
1/1/55–12/31/55	6,742,000	6,692,000	7/1/55–6/30/56		424,299
1/1/56–12/31/56			7/1/56–6/30/57		1,490,853
1/1/57–12/31/57	645,000		7/1/57–6/30/58		1,823,565
1/1/58–12/31/58			7/1/58–6/30/59		1,319,824
1/1/59–12/31/59	500,000		7/1/59–6/30/60	216,750	531,198
1/1/60–12/31/60	1,220,000	720,750	7/1/60–6/30/61	649,000	947,252
1/1/61–12/31/61	22,744,250	912,810	7/1/61–6/30/62	767,810	1,140,640
1/1/62–12/31/62	25,021,441	2,099,370	7/1/62–6/30/63	2,099,370	1,349,513

1/1/63–6/30/64[a]	23,690,938	23,690,938	7/1/63–6/30/64	−198,410	540,751
7/1/64–6/30/65	3,254,063	2,894,063	7/1/64–6/30/65	25,347,170	551,531
7/1/65–6/30/66			7/1/65–6/30/66		8,011,326
7/1/66–6/30/67			7/1/66–6/30/67		6,802,687
7/1/67–6/30/68	8,000,070	8,000,070	7/1/67–6/30/68	8,000,070	5,415,596
7/1/68–6/30/69	1,888,500	1,888,500	7/1/68–6/30/69	1,888,500	4,112,094

Sources: Annual Capital Budgets printed in the *City Record* and the Annual Reports of the Controller of the City of New York.
[a] In 1963 the capital budget was placed on a fiscal-year basis. The period 1/1/63–6/30/64 represents a transitional period of 18 months.

TABLE 4.2

Harlem Hospital Project, Cumulative Data

Date	Budget Adoptions Initiated	Date	Amount Authorized for Expenditure	Actual Expenditures
12/31/52	$ 110,000			
		6/30/53	$ 140,000	$ 27,083
12/31/53	140,000			
		6/30/54	140,000	70,090
12/31/54	140,000			
		6/30/55	6,832,000	148,925
12/31/55	6,832,000			
		6/30/56	6,832,000	573,224
12/31/56	6,832,000			
		6/30/57	6,832,000	2,064,077
12/31/57	6,832,000			
		6/30/58	6,832,000	3,887,642
12/31/58	6,832,000			
		6/30/59	6,832,000	5,207,466
12/31/59	6,832,000			
		6/30/60	7,048,750	5,738,664
12/31/60	7,552,750			
		6/30/61	7,697,750	6,685,916
12/31/61	8,465,560			
		6/30/62	8,465,560	7,826,555
12/31/62[a]	10,564,930			
		6/30/63	10,564,930	9,176,069
6/30/64	34,255,867	6/30/64	10,366,519	9,716,819
6/30/65	37,149,930	6/30/65	35,713,689	10,268,351
6/30/66	37,149,930	6/30/66	35,713,689	18,279,677
6/30/67	37,149,930	6/30/67	35,713,689	25,082,364
6/30/68	45,150,000	6/30/68	43,713,759	30,497,961
6/30/69	47,038,500	6/30/69	45,602,259	34,610,055

Sources: Annual Capital Budgets printed in the *City Record* and the Annual Reports of the Controller of the City of New York.
[a] In 1963 the capital budget was placed on a fiscal-year basis. Adoptions of 12/31/62 were for a transitional 18-month period.

The plans, as filed with the Department of Buildings, called for alterations to the main building and the women's pavilion, and for the construction of a new 200-bed unit on the site of an existing two-story outpatient building. Between 1954 and 1956 the execution of these plans seemed to proceed with little controversy or modification.

Harlem Hospital became something of an issue during the Javits-Wagner senatorial race of 1956. After well-publicized visits to the hospital and meetings with community and political leaders, Mayor Robert Wagner concluded that efforts at renovation were a "waste of money." The physical plant was in undeniably deplorable condition and consultations were started on the feasibility of building a new hospital.

The Draft Capital Budget for 1957, submitted by the City Planning Commission, did not include plans for the construction of a new hospital. The mayor's budget director, in his report to the Board of Estimate, however, recommended the addition of $645,000 for the planning of such a unit. It was reported in the budget that this proposal would raise the estimated total cost of constructing the 200-bed project to $21 million. The Board approved the additional authorization over the objections of the Planning Commission, but subsequently failed to "initiate" the authorization. Thus the funds appeared briefly in the capital budget, were never used, and were removed from the succeeding budget.

The cornerstone-laying ceremony for the 200-bed unit (now known as the "K" building), which had been under construction since 1954, was held during the mayoralty election of 1957. At that ceremony the mayor announced that, in response to the demands of community leaders, he had decided to reconstruct the entire plant. The reconstruction was to take place in three stages. The first step would complete the construction of the "K" building, the cornerstone of which had just been laid. The second, to begin immediately upon completion of the first, would erect a new 500-bed main building. The third stage would see the expansion of the women's pavilion from 271 to 350 beds, and the modernization of the pediatric pavilion.

On the basis of this sequencing of steps, no additional funds were appropriated in 1958, pending the completion of "K" building. During that year, however, community pressure was intensified for speedier action. By late 1958 the "K" building was nearing completion and it was decided to request site acquisition funds for the new main building in the 1959 budget. The selected site was on Lenox Avenue, between 135th and 136th streets, adjacent to the existing structure. Its assessed valuation was $961,000 and approximately 400 families were living on the site.

By the time this decision was reached the Draft Capital Budget had already been prepared by the Planning Commission. The proposal, therefore, again appeared in the budget director's report, which recommended that the Hospital Department's requests be restructured to allow $500,000 for site acquisition and planning for a new building. The Board of Estimate appropriated this amount but, again, failed to "initiate" the expenditure.

In mid-1959 a Harlem group organized a protest against what they considered to be the administration's slow-paced progress. The scheduled opening of "K" building was advanced from September to August, and was held when only parts of the building were ready to admit patients. The formal dedication took place in October, 1959. At the same time the mayor asked for, and received, a resolution from the Board of Estimate approving the selected site for the proposed main building.

Some significant progress was made in 1960. That year's budget contained funds for the project and these were initiated for use. In September preliminary plans were filed with the Department of Buildings and relocation of families living on the site was begun. The 1961 budget included over $22 million for the project construction. Only a portion of these funds was initiated in that year but the total appropriation was repeated in subsequent budgets until the full amount was made available in 1963.

The mayoral election of 1961 again introduced Harlem Hospital's progress as a campaign issue. Delays in construction were emphasized by the opposition, and it was pointed out that as late as August, 1961, there were still some 54 families living on the site.

In 1962 the mayor announced the expansion of the project from

500 to 800 beds. In October groundbreaking ceremonies were held and late in November foundation work began. Work came to a halt in June, 1963, because of the protests of civil rights organizations over low minority-group employment in the construction trades. The unions refused to send workers to the site because of the risk of violent confrontation with picketing protestors. Construction remained at a standstill until November, 1963, when an agreement was reached and the workers returned to the site.

Since that time, work has progressed at what is described as a "normal" pace. A city-wide plumbers' strike, lasting about six months, delayed construction. Some changes in the design have been incorporated as the work progressed: the fifteenth floor, for example, was converted to an intensive care unit and a specialized burn-treatment center was included in the project. The latter was a result of the inclusion of a specialist in the field through the hospital's affiliation contract. Other "normal" delays included changes in hospital and building codes, multiple reviews of all such changes by a variety of agencies, and the "usual" difficulties attendant upon dovetailing the several construction trade activities and inspecting and supervising them. By September, 1969, the main building was ready for dedication by the mayor, and for the appreciative comment of our observer.

Once a hospital is completed, its problems are far from over. There is a need to maintain the facility and provide adequate operating funds to prevent rapid deterioration and obsolescence. Decisions affecting the proper allocation of resources for these purposes are vital aspects of maintaining an effective hospital system. They are, however, outside the scope of this chapter, which is devoted to the management of capital projects.

A MORE FORMAL APPRAISAL
OF THE PROBLEMS

The retrospective view of the Harlem Hospital case has, it is hoped, provided the reader with some sense of the nature and "flavor" of the progress of a capital project in hospital construction. A more formal and analytical view is presented in a recent study by Charlotte Muller and Paul Worthington of the Center for Social Research of the City University of New York. Titled "The Time Structure of Capital Formation: Design and Construction of Municipal Hospital Projects," this study examines the flow of capital expenditures and the progress of twenty-one municipal hospital projects during the twenty-year period of 1946 to 1965. No attempt will be made here to evaluate the methodology or completeness of this study. It represents an analysis of budgeting practices over a twenty-year period, and as such is a useful indicator of the cumulative results of the budgeting practices. Some of the major findings and conclusions of this study are briefly summarized below.

1. Over the twenty-year period under examination, the capital budget adoptions averaged less than two-thirds of the amounts requested by the Department of Hospitals. This is hardly a surprising finding to anyone familiar with any budgeting process. Invariably, it seems one gets less than one asks for. Much more unexpected is the finding that the amount actually spent averaged less than one-half of the amount adopted.

2. Despite the intent of the procedural and legal mechanisms incorporated in the budgeting process, there is no systematic relationship between actual expenditures and adoptions. This holds true even when year-to-year fluctuations are allowed for by considering the cumulative totals. The data show that the time required for cumulative expenditures to match adoptions has increased substantially in the past twenty years. In 1948, cumulative expenditures were equal to cumulative adoptions of a year earlier. By 1965, however, cumulative expenditures just equaled cumulative adoptions in 1953—a lag of twelve years.

3. Since there is a huge backlog of adoptions and expenditures, the study points out that one cannot conclude that a limitation of borrowing power rations the construction of capital improvements. The frequently heard claim that the plant and equipment of the municipal system are inefficient and of poor quality because they have been starved for funds simply does not hold up. The funds

are "there," they are adoptions in the budget. Although Muller and Worthington say quality is poor *not* for lack of capital funds, the hospitals may well be starved for operating funds. This lack may produce the rapid deterioration, obsolescence, and dilapidation which characterize municipal facilities.

4. The length of time required to implement a project is *not* proportional to its size, as might be expected. Using a project's dollar value as a measure of its size, one finds that time does *not* increase in the same proportion as cost. Higher-cost projects take longer to complete than lower-cost ones, but not proportionately longer. It should be noted that "project duration," as measured in this study, begins with actual design process and ends when the project is reported as at 95 percent completion. Excluded from this "project duration" is the time spent on site selection as well as on all capital allocation and budgeting procedures which precede the design phase. It is suspected that, when the periods of time spent on these activities are added to the project duration, its length would prove even *less* proportional to the magnitude of the project.

5. The time taken by the design stage constitutes about half the total time required for project completion. That is to say, design time averages just a trifle less than construction time for all projects, and this relationship obtains regardless of the size of the project. Furthermore, economies of scale with respect to time tend to be less evident in the design activity than in the construction activity. As *total* time requirements increase, time requirements for *design* increase proportionately *more* than time requirements for construction.

The Muller-Worthington study identifies some specific legal and administrative practices of New York City which contribute to the patterns identified above. It is perhaps useful to introduce at this stage a number of basic notions drawn from more generalized administrative models. These notions explain the findings of the Muller-Worthington study in broader managerial terms, which need not rely on factors peculiar to New York City or to hospital design and construction. This broader interpretation should be useful in opening up a wider perspective and framework within which remedies and improvements can be sought and developed.

TWO MODELS FROM MANAGEMENT SCIENCE

In recent years, Management Science (or Operations Research) has advanced the application of mathematics and symbolic model building to the analysis and solution of administrative and logistic problems. Rigorous mathematical analyses have shed light on many phases of business and industrial operations with, perhaps, foremost emphasis given to problems of logistics and adaptation to changing constraints.

Without introducing any of the quantitative elements involved, it is useful here to refer briefly to two such models. Both, it should be noted, are "dynamic" models in their explicit consideration of changes over time. The first comes out of the work of Jay Forrester of MIT in the field which he named "Industrial Dynamics." Forrester focuses on the time dimension and its impact on the operations of a business. At the risk of oversimplifying a complex mathematical analysis, we can state that Forrester's work traces the effects of the time lag inherent in any administrative response to change. Even as simple an operation as ordering the production of goods in response to the placement of customer orders is discovered to generate a series of fluctuations in the system, the magnitude and direction of which are largely determined by the time lags built into the system.

Forrester has shown that any lengthening of the time between the receipt of the input signal (e.g., the customer's order) and its execution by the organization amplifies the fluctuations involved, reduces the effectiveness of the response, and increases the disparity between input information and the outputs actually delivered by the system. Moreover, these distortions are shown to result directly from the increased *time lag*, without regard to the magnitudes involved in the process or the complexity of the procedures causing the time lag. A secondary factor contributing to the distortion of response is found in the *frequency of changes* in the input signal, again without direct regard to the nature of the process or the procedures involved.

Applying this notion to the findings of the Muller-Worthington hospital study, we see that it is apparent why no obvious, systematic link is found between adoptions (input signals) and expenditures (outputs). The extensive time lag built into the capital budgeting

Figure 4.1. New York City Capital Budget Adoptions and Expenditures for Health and Hospital Facilities, 1951-1968

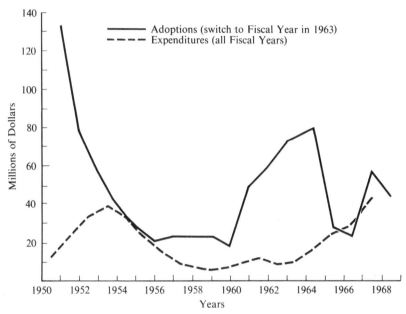

Source: See Tables 4.3 and 4.4.

and implementation cycle, itself, tends to distort such linkages, despite the legal and procedural framework's intent to keep the two in balance. Equally evident is the fact that frequent changes in the input signal, such as exemplified the changes and reverses described in the Harlem Hospital case, reinforce the tendency to distort the relation between inputs and outputs. That this does in fact happen is illustrated by Figure 4.1, which presents capital budget adoptions and expenditures over a seventeen-year period.

One can discern no stable pattern or systematic relationship between the inputs (adoptions) and the outputs (expenditures). The fluctuations would be even more extreme if we included the immediate postwar period (1946–50), which experienced large budget adoptions.

TABLE 4.3

Yearly Capital Budget Adoptions for Health and Hospitals Departments (in thousands of dollars)

Year	Amount	Percent of Total Budget
1951	.$134,199	32.3
1952	77,015	16.0
1953	57,225	15.0
1954	38,067	8.2
1955	29,484	4.2
1956	21,583	3.6
1957	23,689	4.3
1958	23,290	4.1
1959	23,776	4.3
1960	17,062	2.9
1961	49,042	8.1
1962	59,886	7.0
1963–64[a]	73,211	7.2
1964–65	79,674	10.1
1965–66	27,860	4.7
1966–67	24,168	4.5
1967–68	57,018	8.4
1968–69	45,478	7.4

Source: Data supplied by Capital Budget Division, City Planning Commission.
[a] 18 months.

The Forrester model further demonstrates the distortions in project duration when measured against project size. Since almost all the procedural time lags built into the system are independent of the size of the project, their impact and distorting influences apply almost equally to high-cost and low-cost projects alike. Once a project is defined as a capital budget item, the procedural steps prescribed for its processing are not affected by its dollar value.

Chart 4.1 readily indicates the many steps and agencies involved in the procedure. This chart is a somewhat simplified representation of reality and was prepared by the Mayor's Task Force on Urban Design. The forty-nine steps shown do not include a series of prescribed public hearings, required reviews with the Health and Hospital Planning Council, and the many informal consultations and reviews interspersed at various stages of the formal process. Built-in

TABLE 4.4

Yearly Capital Budget Expenditures for Health and Hospital Facilities

Fiscal Year	Amount	Fiscal Year	Amount
1950–51	$13,737,450	1959-60	$6,942,883
1951–52	24,305,833	1960-61	9,705,357
1952–53	34,432,403	1961-62	12,984,625
1953–54	39,673,247	1962-63	9,330,243
1954–55	34,673,435	1963-64	10,224,322
1955–56	23,520,519	1964-65	17,518,591
1956–57	15,447,096	1965-66	26,107,598
1957–58	9,787,596	1966-67	29,648,999
1958–59	7,366,606	1967-68	43,328,636

Source: Annual Reports of the Controller, Part 3, Statement 4.

time lags are equally numerous during the construction phase of the project, involving inspections, acceptances, payment approvals, etc. These, too, are largely independent of the size of the project.

The Forrester model also demonstrates another finding of the Muller-Worthington study: the design stage of the process is affected by both changes in the input signal and built-in time lags. One can realistically assume that the frequency of changes in the input signal is higher in the design phase than it is in the construction stage. This assumption will readily explain the greater distortions (and reduced economies of scale) in the designing of projects than in their construction. Once changes in signal are introduced, a variety of procedural steps are prescribed for the review and approval of planning changes. Thus frequency in signal change and time lags

CHART 4. 1. MAYOR'S TASK FORCE ON URBAN DESIGN:

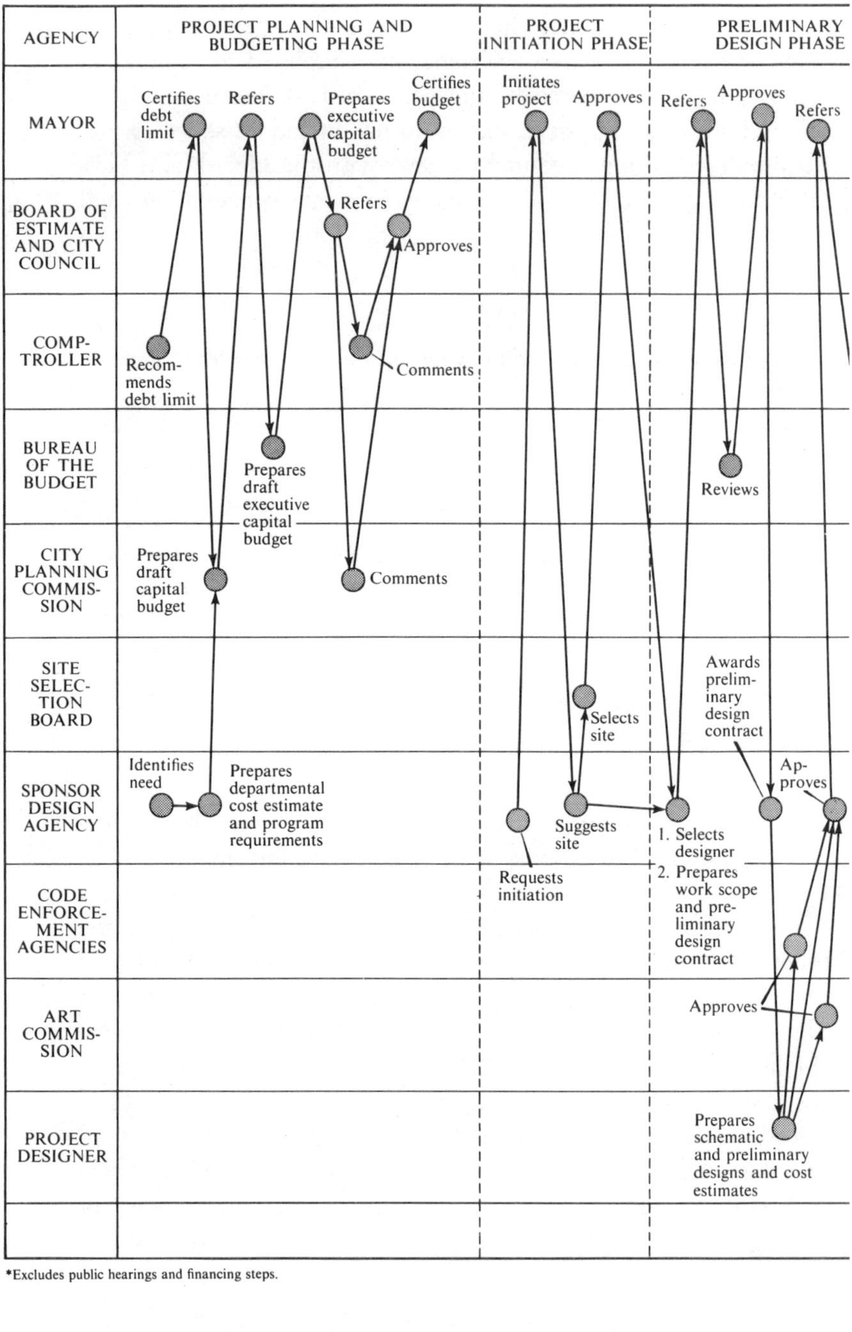

AGENCY	PROJECT PLANNING AND BUDGETING PHASE	PROJECT INITIATION PHASE	PRELIMINARY DESIGN PHASE
MAYOR	Certifies debt limit — Refers — Prepares executive capital budget — Certifies budget	Initiates project — Approves	Refers — Approves — Refers
BOARD OF ESTIMATE AND CITY COUNCIL	Refers — Approves		
COMPTROLLER	Recommends debt limit — Comments		
BUREAU OF THE BUDGET	Prepares draft executive capital budget		Reviews
CITY PLANNING COMMISSION	Prepares draft capital budget — Comments		
SITE SELECTION BOARD		Selects site	Awards preliminary design contract
SPONSOR DESIGN AGENCY	Identifies need — Prepares departmental cost estimate and program requirements	Suggests site	1. Selects designer 2. Prepares work scope and preliminary design contract — Approves
CODE ENFORCEMENT AGENCIES		Requests initiation	
ART COMMISSION			Approves
PROJECT DESIGNER			Prepares schematic and preliminary designs and cost estimates

*Excludes public hearings and financing steps.

EXISTING PROCEDURES FOR CAPITAL PROJECT DEVELOPMENT*

	FINAL DESIGN PHASE			CONTRACT DOCUMENTS PHASE			CONSTRUCTION PHASE	NUMBER OF ACTIONS
Ap-proves	Refers Approves Approves Refers							14
								2
								2
Re-views	Reviews	Reviews						5
								2
				Adver-tises for bids	Analyzes bids	Awards four con-struction contracts		1
	Awards contract	Approves		Prepares bid docu-ments (four contracts)	Receives bids	Reviews bidder qualifi-cations	Supervises construction	17
	1. Selects designer 2. Prepares work scope and final design contract							2
	Approves	Approves						2
		Prepares final designs and cost estimate						2
						TOTAL		49

combine to stretch out that part of the process most directly affected by changes in planning—the design stage. This elongation may, in turn, invite subsequent signal changes.

The second management science model which we will consider explains the large and growing backlog of appropriations noted in the Muller-Worthington study. It is generally referred to as a "Queuing Model" and is an important segment of queuing or waiting-line theories. This model examines the behavior of a typical servicing center or system: units arrive at certain rates, they are processed or serviced, and then they depart from the system. It has been extensively used in such applications as tollbooths on bridges, planes landing at airports, or customers arriving at a store counter. The model permits the prediction of such characteristics of the system as the length of the queue, the probability of idle service time, and the average waiting time in line. The reasoning can be readily extended to the capital budgeting process. Here appropriations represent the arriving units, completed projects the departing units, and the backlog of unspent appropriations the queue or backup in the pipeline.

Again without regard to the mathematics involved, the queuing model points up a number of conclusions, some of which are obvious and others less so. It is, for example, rather obvious that if the rate of arrivals is the same as the rate of departures the only way a queue can be avoided (or kept at a constant level) is by the precise scheduling of arrivals and of each servicing time to match the departures. Not as obvious is the significant impact created by the introduction of randomness in the pattern of either arrivals, servicing time, or departures, even when their *average* rate of arrival remains constant. Customers, for example, may arrive at a counter at an average rate of 10 per hour, but these 10 arrivals might be spread at random throughout the hour—3 customers in the first 10 minutes, 5 more in the next 45 minutes, and the remaining 2 in the last 5 minutes. Similarly, the servicing of customers can vary from, say, 2 minutes to 10 minutes, while the average rate of departures can be a constant 10 per hour.

Once such randomness is introduced in either arrivals or departures, a large queue or backlog can be prevented only by providing for a processing capacity significantly larger than would be necessary to service the average rate of arrivals. Otherwise, as the processing (or departures) rate approaches the rate of arrivals, the length of the queue rises sharply. Mathematically, it can be demonstrated that the queue will be infinite when service rate equals arrivals rate.

If we translate these concepts into the capital budgeting process, it becomes evident that the administrative goal of balancing appropriations (arrivals) with expenditures (departures) *must* result in a growing backlog of unspent funds if there is any degree of randomness at either end of the pipeline (even if processing time is assumed to be relatively constant).

Any unforeseen delay in design, construction, or even in payments on work done introduces randomness in the system's output, while the addition of appropriations without a clear and sequenced plan for their use introduces randomness at the input. The Harlem Hospital case history suggests that a considerable amount of variation at both ends of the pipeline must be expected in any capital project and that construction funds are allocated in irregular amounts over several years. The more random the arrivals and departures (at the highly critical end of the scale where these are expected to be nearly equal), the longer the waiting line, the faster it grows, and the lower the ratio of actual expenditures to backlog.

The Muller-Worthington findings of a growing backlog of appropriated but unspent funds represent the lengthening queue which the model predicts. As this queue lengthens with increased variations between inputs and outputs, it is not surprising to find that actual expenditures become a smaller percentage of cumulative total appropriations. Expenditures can decrease even to the point, noted in the study, where they represent less than 50 percent of appropriations. In fact, the queuing model predicts that unless variations from plan (in both inputs and outputs) are reduced, the backlog may keep growing indefinitely.

The review of these two administrative models suggests that *any* logistic system will exhibit the kind of distortions pointed out in the Muller-Worthington study and often bemoaned by critics of the city's capital project programs. There is nothing uniquely evil in this system. It displays the same characteristics as other administrative systems, and can be improved by modifying these characteristics. The two models, further, permit the identification of those factors which are the primary determinants of the distortions noted.

It may prove comforting to note that the determinants are obvious. Less obvious, perhaps, is the conclusion that three relatively simple characteristics account for a great variety of administrative ailments and symptoms. Our examination of the two models suggests that, in the administrative system, the extent and magnitude of distortions depend upon three primary characteristics of the system: (1) the number and frequency of changes in input signals or plans, (2) the extent of time lags built into the system, and (3) the degree of unforeseen randomness or deviation from planned time schedules.

In the balance of this chapter we will identify the presence and relative importance of each of these three distortion-causing characteristics at each phase of the hospital construction process. We will then point up some suggestions for reducing their magnitude and negative impact.

MANAGING THE DYNAMICS OF
CAPITAL PROJECTS

The long and complex path from idea to completed structure is best analyzed by dividing it into four distinct phases, at least conceptually. Phase 1 may be titled *policy formulation*. This is the phase which determines the general posture and strategy of municipal health services and selects specific projects as appropriate undertakings within that over-all strategy. It includes the clarifying of objectives, purposes, and missions of the city's efforts in health services; the meshing of municipal and voluntary programs; the allocation of resources (in block sums) to major programs; and the spelling out of the broad specifications of mission and scope of an individual project. This phase typically concludes with the recommendation to seek a capital appropriation for selected projects.

Phase 2 consists of *capital budgeting*. This phase is primarily, but not entirely, procedural. It involves the process which results in specific budget appropriations for each subsequent phase of a capital project. There are many prescribed procedural steps to be followed, but issues of substance also get resolved in the process. Any differences of opinion among the Hospital Department, the Planning Commission, the Bureau of the Budget, and other agencies involved are ironed out in the process of determining appropriations.

Phase 3 can be described as *technical planning* and is largely concerned with the architectural and facility design. Plans for buildings, equipment, and supporting facilities are drawn up and taken through various stages of examination and approval.

Phase 4 is the *construction* stage and involves the physical implementation of all the plans, including inspection and approval of the steps leading to the acceptance of a completed building.

Having identified the four phases of the process, we can now proceed to examine the distortion-causing characteristics peculiar to each phase and suggest approaches for their control.

Phase 1: The Dynamics of Policy Formulation

It is at this phase in the process that the broadest issues and the most diversified constituencies must be considered and integrated. Political, social, and community forces must be meshed with financial constraints, professional demands, and the efforts of other sectors. Some notion of the diversity of interests involved in forging an over-all strategy for municipal health services can be obtained by considering some of the major forces involved. The mission and functions of the municipal hospital system must be fulfilled against this background. The needs of the consumer of health services and his ability to pay place certain demands on the total system. Organizations of consumer groups and community and political pressures on elected officials serve to supplement and modify these needs. The resources made available for any program depend on the availability of federal, state, and local governmental funds, as well as health insurance programs, whether governmental or private.

The medical and allied health professions, as well as the technology involved, impose major constraints on the kind and extent of services to be offered. The relative priority placed on other-than-health programs obviously makes competing demands on the limited resources available. Similarly the professional and administrative philosophies of the senior officials in charge inevitably guide and shape the strategies that have been formulated.

In terms of the administrative characteristics of this phase of the process, the greatest danger is posed by the first of the distortions we identified, namely, the changes, reversals, and modifications of the "input signals" into the subsequent phases. Changes in political or community aspirations and a mayor's response to them can make significant alterations in the over-all strategy of health services. Equally significant are the implications of such federal and state programs as Medicare and Medicaid. Yet in the face of such fluctuations it remains essential to maintain a unified direction and thrust in long-run policy and to originate a relatively consistent set of signals to actuate the subsequent phases of the capital project process. It must be realized that hospital buildings take about seven years or more to erect, and they are amortized over several decades thereafter, while mayors are elected to four-year terms and hospital commissioners may be replaced at even shorter intervals.

If relative stability of input signal is to be maintained, two criteria must be achieved. The first requirement is a suitable mechanism for resolving and integrating conflicting and fluctuating external forces. In the past, local communities have often had to react to proposals long after their initial formulation. Depending upon the power of their organization and their connections with political leadership these local groups may have been able to force modifications late in the construction process. A more satisfactory mechanism would incorporate representatives to voice the communities' sentiments in the initial policy formulation stage. Second, these fluctuations and conflicts should be insulated, as far as possible, from the subsequent phases of the process. Implied in both factors is the need for a reasonably stable, consistent, and long-range strategy which is responsive to, but is not overwhelmed by, any one of the forces competing for attention.

The recent recognition of a city-sponsored Organizational Task Force under a federal comprehensive health-planning statute presents a unique opportunity to achieve the two desired criteria.

Approved by the New York State Health Department, the Organizational Task Force has the responsibility to design the structure for the planning mechanism for the city's health services. The final design should provide for a forum in which all constituencies can be heard and considered, a forum in which economic, political, and social factors are presented and debated. The mechanism should also, however, place heavy emphasis on the evolution of a stable, consistent strategy and the insulation of short-run conflicts from the input signals which initiate specific projects within that over-all strategy. The prospects for an effective policy formulation mechanism are much better than recent experience might indicate. The Health and Hospital Planning Council of Southern New York, which was envisioned as performing essentially the same function, was largely oriented to the voluntary hospital sector, and although it expressed judgments on municipal health budgets and projects, it was less instrumental in integrating municipal programs. The newly designed mechanism should better integrate both sectors and at the same time be responsive to the several constituencies represented in policy formulation.

If a consistency of input signal is achieved in this phase, the impact of the two remaining administrative characteristics becomes of secondary importance. Time lags and deviations from planned schedules need not cause any distortions in the remaining phases of the process once policy formulation is effectively insulated from them. The machinery of budgeting, design, and construction is, in effect, not activated until an input signal emerges from the policy formulation phase. Activities preceding that signal are thus excluded from the remaining steps of the capital budgeting process.

Phase 2: The Dynamics of Capital Budgeting

Reference has already been made to the elaborate, multistepped procedures embodied in the city's capital budgeting process. In Chart 4.1 these steps are shown under the headings of "Project Planning and Budgeting Phase" and "Project Initiation Phase." We also noted that many formal procedural steps are taken only after much informal consultation and negotiation between agencies and officials. Considerable time may elapse in this phase of the process. Although amendments are possible throughout the year, the fact that capital budgeting proceeds according to statutory deadlines means that when the preparatory work cannot be completed by the due date action is frequently delayed. At other times the preparation is rushed to meet deadlines and its quality, accuracy, or reliability suffers as a result.

In terms of our administrative model, this phase of the process can best be improved by (a) reducing time lags built into the system and (b) reducing the degree of variation between the appropriation fed into the pipeline and the expenditures flowing out of it.

The most effective way of reducing time lags is to reduce the number of prescribed steps in the process and, if possible, the number of agencies involved in it. A specific procedure-simplification recommendation is beyond the scope of this chapter. The recommendation that this be done is not. We note that the Mayor's Task Force on Urban Design did propose such simplifications, and these are represented in Chart 4.2. Without discussing the specific merits of the proposed procedure, we can endorse its objectives. The Task Force combines the first two phases of Chart 4.1 into a single phase, titled "Planning and Budgeting Phase." It reduces the number of steps shown from eighteen to eight, and the number of agencies involved from seven to six. Both trends are highly desirable in terms of our model.

It may, perhaps, be useful to add a word about the intent and focus of procedural steps, quite aside from their number. Too often municipal procedures focus almost exclusively on the prevention of petty theft or malpractice. While these must, of course, be guarded against, they cannot be regarded as the sole reasons for established procedure. The efficiency and effectiveness of the process must also receive full attention. There are too many examples of governmental procedures which succeed in preventing a $5 theft at the cost of $100,000 of waste or oversight.

The second improvement to be pursued in this phase should seek to achieve a better balance between inputs (appropriations) and outputs (expenditures). The alarming expansion of the budgetary backlog as a result of poor balancing has already been noted. It needs to be emphasized, however, that a growing backlog of unspent

CHART 4. 2. MAYOR'S TASK FORCE ON URBAN DESIGN: RECOMMENDED PROCEDURES FOR CAPITAL PROJECT DEVELOPMENT*

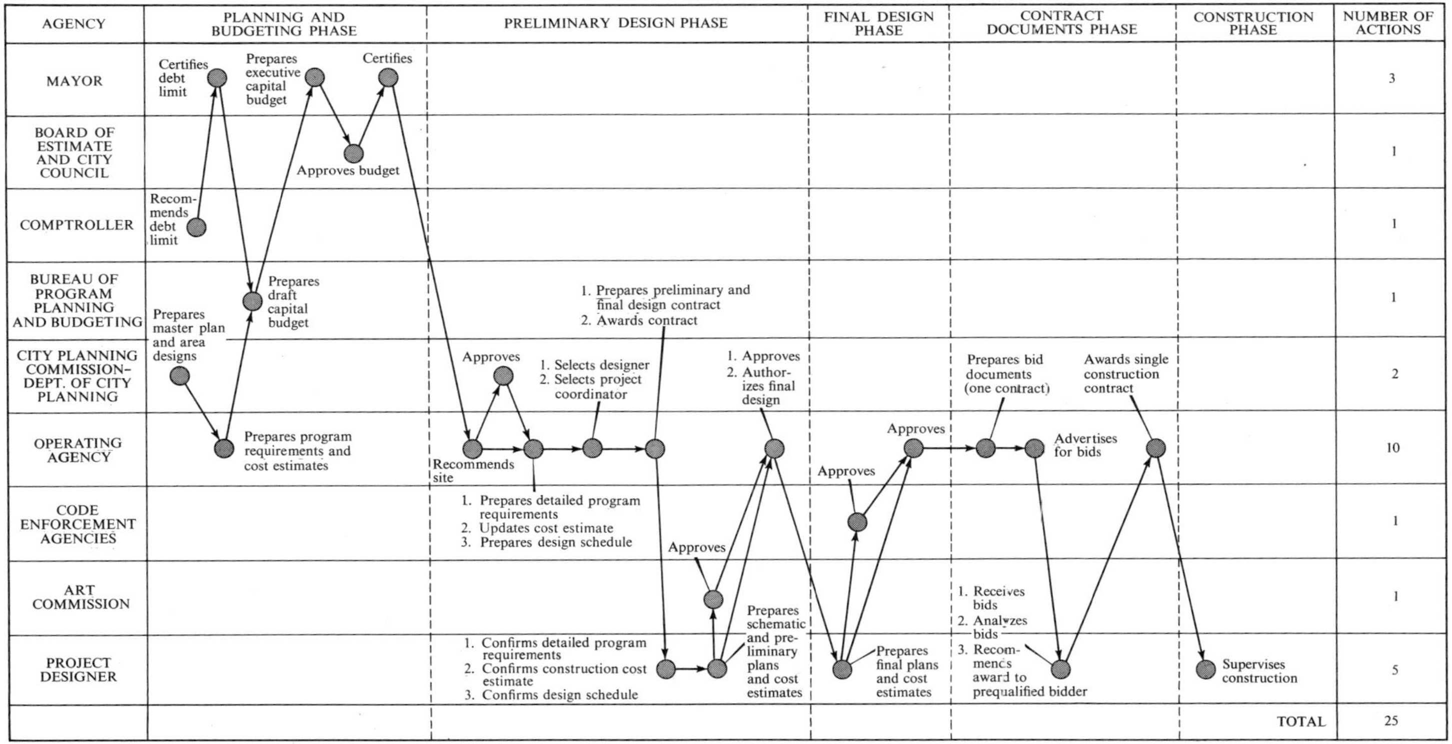

AGENCY	PLANNING AND BUDGETING PHASE	PRELIMINARY DESIGN PHASE	FINAL DESIGN PHASE	CONTRACT DOCUMENTS PHASE	CONSTRUCTION PHASE	NUMBER OF ACTIONS
MAYOR	Certifies debt limit — Prepares executive capital budget — Certifies					3
BOARD OF ESTIMATE AND CITY COUNCIL	Approves budget					1
COMPTROLLER	Recommends debt limit					1
BUREAU OF PROGRAM PLANNING AND BUDGETING	Prepares draft capital budget					1
CITY PLANNING COMMISSION-DEPT. OF CITY PLANNING	Prepares master plan and area designs	1. Prepares preliminary and final design contract 2. Awards contract				2
OPERATING AGENCY	Prepares program requirements and cost estimates	Recommends site — Approves — 1. Selects designer 2. Selects project coordinator — 1. Approves 2. Authorizes final design	Approves — Approves			10
CODE ENFORCEMENT AGENCIES		Approves				1
ART COMMISSION			Approves			1
PROJECT DESIGNER		1. Prepares detailed program requirements 2. Updates cost estimate 3. Prepares design schedule — Prepares schematic and preliminary plans and cost estimates — 1. Confirms detailed program requirements 2. Confirms construction cost estimate 3. Confirms design schedule	Prepares final plans and cost estimates	Prepares bid documents (one contract) — Advertises for bids — 1. Receives bids 2. Analyzes bids 3. Recommends award to prequalified bidder — Awards single construction contract	Supervises construction	5
					TOTAL	25

*Excludes public hearings and financing steps.

appropriations is objectionable not only from the aesthetic point of view. As the Muller-Worthington study points out, unspent appropriations use up a scarce resource—the city's debt capacity. The "leaner" the backlog in the budget, the more flexibility there is for the city administration to allocate its financial resources.

Better phasing of inputs and outputs can be achieved by keeping closer track of work completion and by more accurate forecasting of the expenditures which will actually be made in the coming fiscal year. These improvements, in turn, can be achieved by centralizing and coordinating information flows, and by use of such techniques as PERT, the Critical Path Method, and the many variants of these. The recent creation of a specialized section in the Bureau of the Budget and the information system being designed for it are clearly steps in the right direction.

We might also add here that the insulation of policy formulation from budgeting operations proposed in the preceding section should contribute to the closer matching of inputs and outputs. The mechanism for setting priorities in Phase 1 should, it is hoped, provide the mayor with a forum for demonstrating his concern for a program by means other than a large appropriation in the current budget. The addition of such appropriations simply as an indication of sympathy for a given program (whether or not such appropriations are subsequently utilized) only serves to broaden the gulf between appropriations and expenditures.

Phase 3: The Dynamics of Technical Planning

The architect, the designer, and the engineer become the focal point of this phase of the process. A hospital building represents a complex blending of provision for patient needs, structural design, special-purpose space and manpower utilization, provision for elaborate equipment installation, and aesthetic consideration. The task is a time-consuming one and, as noted in the Muller-Worthington study, takes almost as long as the final construction phase. In terms of our administrative model, undue stretch-outs are the result of two characteristics: changes in input signal and built-in time lags. These will be examined in sequence.

It is quite obvious that changes in mission and scope of services, as well as in technical specifications, set off an elaborate series of modifications in the design work once it has been launched. Changes in scope and mission originate primarily in Phase 1—policy formulation. Our review of the Harlem Hospital case indicates the impact on design time of the decision to increase bed capacity from 500 to 800 and to add a burn-treatment facility.

While some modification in mission and scope is probably inevitable, many fluctuations can be avoided by greater consistency in planning resulting from a longer-run, stable strategy for health services. The importance of a consistent strategy has already been emphasized in our discussion of Phase 1. It is necessary only to point out the beneficial results of such consistency on the technical planning phase.

A second major factor responsible for changes in input signal at this phase is technological change. Continuous advances in the state of the art of medicine and its technology reflect directly on the design of hospital structures and facilities. In the designer's efforts to incorporate the latest advances and to avoid the creation of an obsolete structure he faces the prospect of almost continuous modifications. This is a serious problem, but is not unique to hospital construction. The aircraft and aerospace industries face this issue in almost every project.

The approach employed by these industries must, in the final analysis, be adopted here too. Designers must accept the fact that they *cannot* adopt every technical innovation as it occurs. A stage is reached in the design process when the technology is "frozen." Further modification is ruled out and the project is implemented. To do otherwise would mean that a high-technology project would *never* be completed.

Coupled with the acceptance of an inevitable obsolescence is the approach that says designers should retain flexibility as far into the construction stage as possible. This approach has been suggested for hospital construction. Prominent hospital architects have argued for the design of structures which permit considerable variation in space allocation and equipment addition even after the basic shell has been completed. The adoption of this approach to design would significantly reduce the number and extent of planning changes, with direct benefits to both the technical design phase and the construction phase. It also encourages the kind of construction which permits more flexible uses of the structure over its lifetime.

As mentioned earlier, technical planning is also affected by built-in time lags. Prescribed approvals of each type of design change require multiagency consideration of many (and often minor) alterations in plans. Each of these becomes time consuming as the approving agencies find their work load increasing in the face of limited resources of skilled and competent manpower.

The extended design period for hospital projects is occasionally blamed on the architects' and consultants' reluctance to assign high priorities to city projects. We do not find this argument persuasive or convincing. It is true that some technical firms are reluctant to undertake work for the city, citing "red tape" and frustration as their chief reasons. Those who do, however, have no incentive to delay or prolong the design project. Consulting firms, in any field, fare best when work on hand is completed as rapidly as possible. Since design work is paid for by the size of the project rather than by the time expended, there is no obvious economic incentive for delay or "stretch-out."

The key to accelerating technical planning lies in improving the administrative characteristics we have noted: decreasing changes in signals, retaining flexibility for technological change, and reducing administrative time lags. Little, if any, improvement can result from expecting the designers to "work faster."

Phase 4: The Dynamics of Construction

Construction of large, complex buildings is a slow, time-consuming process under the best of conditions. It is aggravated, in municipal hospital projects, by each of the three administrative characteristics we have been tracing. The third, deviation from schedules, however, is by far the most important.

Once construction has begun, changes in planning inputs can obviously cause considerable and costly delays. Such changes, however, typically originate in earlier phases and are not by-products of the construction stage itself. The recommendations made earlier, especially in relation to the policy-formulating and technical-planning phases, would largely alleviate the change-of-signals problems in construction.

Built-in time lags present a more direct problem in this phase. Construction advances subject to a large number of prescribed procedural steps for approvals, inspections, and audits at different stages of the process. A variety of city agencies may be involved and many of them are called upon to service a broad range of programs and projects. The Department of Public Works, for example, is charged with *all* municipal construction and could well find itself torn between the conflicting priorities of hospitals, schools, and subway building projects. Even with the best of intentions, it cannot be completely responsive to the inevitable emergencies and crash-programs which arise in any construction program.

Inspection and supervision of completed work stages often cause delays and, at times, added costs. Apparent shortages in competent manpower are reflected in the tendency of agencies to attempt to add to their own supervisory staffs to meet their work load or to contract the supervision out to private firms. The former procedure does not really solve the problem of manpower shortage for city agencies as a whole, although it may increase the responsiveness of inspectors to their agency's needs.

The attempts at contracting-out seem to provide a genuine solution. The practice of engaging a "third party" supervisor, however, is rather unusual and needs to be questioned. The normal practice in private construction is to retain the building's designers or architects as supervisors. They are most familiar with the project's specifications and have a genuine interest in seeing them carried out effectively. It would seem sensible to adopt the same practice in municipal construction rather than to introduce a new layer of supervision into the already complicated relationship between designer and building contractor. We suspect that any cost savings in the latter arrangement are largely illusory.

The most severe impact of the construction phase on the over-all capital projects process, however, is introduced by deviations from planned time schedules. All construction work is subject to unforeseen deviations: strikes, material shortages, labor availability, and even weather changes. As these factors delay planned schedules, the budgeter's efforts to balance appropriations and expenditures are frustrated, with the results already noted. In the case of municipal construction the probability of wider deviations is substantially increased by the statutory requirement of four separate contractors for all projects. In addition to a general building contractor, three separate contracts must be let: for plumbing, heating and ventilation, and electrical work.

In the absence of a single manager of the total project, the difficulties of coordinating and meshing the work of the several trades involved are seriously magnified. Progress in one area depends upon completion of earlier stages in another, and this interdependence requires a high order of cooperation and close communication. The same interdependence makes it difficult to pinpoint the true cause of delays or errors. This situation is greatly aggravated by the diffusion of authority and responsibility among four independent contractors.

Consideration should be given to some revision of the statute, with a view to permitting a single authority to be in charge, even if the arrangement of four separate bids is to be retained. Alternatively, the same results could be achieved by the use of public or state corporations which could consolidate and integrate many of the interagency and intercontractor jurisdictions. This approach has been taken in the creation of the State Dormitory Authority for Higher Education, and it has been introduced in the State Health and Mental Hygiene Facilities Improvement Corporation.

A ready parallel can be drawn. The establishment of the Health and Hospitals Corporation was designed to remove the many details involved in the day-to-day *operations* of a hospital from an already overburdened and procedurally restricted city administration. There are also many complexities inherent in the *construction* of the city administration's facilities. The basic philosophy of delegating or contracting out specialized and complex tasks, whether to private or public authorities, promises relief to municipal agencies as well as improved task efficiency.

CONCLUSION

In summary, the path of municipal hospital construction is indeed a long and tortuous one. Much of it is inherent in the nature of, and the complexities implied in, the two words "municipal" and "hospital." The extent of delays, distortions, and waste along the path can, however, be reduced. We have argued for the recognition of certain dynamic characteristics common to all administrative processes that are largely responsible for the observed deficiencies. We have further attempted to indicate the relative importance of these characteristics in the different phases of capital project development and have suggested approaches to improved system design.

Our identification of certain "universal" characteristics in all administrative processes, however, must not be pushed too far. We recognize that major and important constraints are introduced when government, rather than private business, is charged with the administrative responsibility. Both sectors, admittedly, face a complex environment and a multitude of conflicting interests and constituencies. In the case of government, however, the demands of such constituencies are more diverse, while the authority to act is more dispersed and subject to greater externally imposed constraints. Government cannot operate with the same ease of flexibility as a business corporation. It would be naïve to believe that it can.

On the other hand, the lessons learned in the management of corporate enterprise and the very existence of the business sector cannot be ignored in dealing with governmental problems. This axiom underlies the arguments presented in this chapter. Improvements in the management of municipal capital projects can be achieved by applying business techniques and approaches, as well as by making better use of the resources and flexibility of the business sector.

In the juxtaposing of business and government, our recommendations can be broadly classified in three categories. First, wherever possible, it is imperative to insulate the purely administrative processes from the political and governmental forces which contribute the main differences between "government" and "business."

This would make the administrative procedure more analogous to independent business and would permit the application of its approaches and techniques. We are not arguing for the *elimination* of the complexities and conflicts inherent in governmental policy formulation, which would be highly undesirable even if it were feasible. We are arguing, however, for a mechanism which would prevent the administrative process from being buffeted about by each shift in an ongoing public debate and would insulate it from the relative momentary standing of diverse political forces. No administrative machinery can function effectively if it responds to every momentary shift in the winds of social or political debate.

Secondly, we argue that wherever administrative processes resemble those encountered in business, full use should be made of managerial attitudes and techniques developed in that sector. Several suggestions under this heading have been presented. These include the need for procedure simplification, the use of modern planning tools and information systems, as well as approaches to coping with technological change and multicontract coordination. A significant body of knowledge and experience has been accumulated by corporate managers in these areas that is highly amenable to governmental application, as has been amply demonstrated by NASA and the Department of Defense. It is not entirely coincidental that business executives are so often invited to participate as trustees, commissioners, or advisers to a large variety of institutions in the field of health services.

Finally, we argue for making greater use of the business sector itself, and the comparative freedom it enjoys vis-à-vis government. The use of private or public corporations as relatively independent "contractors" is a long-established practice. It has, in recent years, been extended to the operation and construction of such governmental projects as schools. It can be applied further in such areas as design, coordination, and inspection of construction in progress for structures as specialized and complex as a modern hospital.

The recent creation of an Organizational Task Force for a comprehensive health-planning agency presents a unique opportunity for improving the effectiveness of the management of capital projects. The administrative concepts and suggestions presented in this chapter (as well as the broader framework presented in this volume) should, it is hoped, provide sound guidelines for the design job ahead. There is little doubt that the administrative characteristics designed into the system, as presented here, will have crucial impacts on the dynamics of capital project development in health services.

5

AFFILIATION CONTRACTS

MUNICIPAL HOSPITAL–UNIVERSITY affiliations in New York City are not new. In fact, an association of Bellevue Hospital and the College of Physicians and Surgeons was established as early as the eighteenth century. As other major medical schools developed in the city, similar agreements were forged linking municipal facilities with one or more universities for teaching purposes. These faculty-staffed hospitals constituted the elite of the municipal system, and Bellevue, for one, achieved international renown.

But not until 1961, when the Commissioner of Hospitals undertook the bold step of contracting through the use of tax funds for the provision of medical staff by private institutions to all the city hospitals upon which the indigent depend for care, did affiliation assume significance as a public policy issue. Since then it has become the key instrument for change in the vast city health complex. The importance of affiliation lies less in its current operations and accomplishments than in the direction it sets for control, operation, regulation, and standard-setting of the increasingly expensive tax-subsidized (pluralistic) medical care system in the city.

The genesis of the current affiliation system reveals the lag between recognition of a problem in municipal services and programmatic responses. There are major obstacles to intervention that is aimed at basic changes in an ongoing system of public service except when there is deterioration to the point of imminent collapse. In the area of shared (public-private) services, the city is impotent to move unless there is clear mutual advantage.

New York is not the only metropolis whose public hospitals

have been affiliated with teaching institutions. In Boston, a long relationship has existed between Boston City Hospital and Harvard, Tufts, and Boston universities; in Chicago a similar loose affiliation has been in effect for many years between Cook County Hospital and the University of Illinois. The affiliation system in New York City is unique, however, because of the scale of the municipal hospital operation and the fact that affiliation represents a reversal of historic municipal policy whereby the city operated its own hospital services for the indigent. The new pattern of affiliations is noteworthy because it has evolved simultaneously with the extraordinary infusion since World War II of tax funds into the production of health services and the explicit assumption by the federal government of broader responsibility for medical care, medical research, and, covertly, medical education. Finally, the affiliation system has suggested to critics and to proponents alike the necessity for some resolution of the gross imbalances that continue to characterize the two segments of hospital care, public and voluntary, in New York City.

What precisely is the affiliation system? In this discussion, it refers specifically to the policy instituted by the Commissioner of Hospitals, in 1961, of contracting with selected teaching and "strong" voluntary hospitals to staff specific municipal hospitals with medical and technical personnel under budgetary terms covering salaries, a percentage for overhead, and some equipment and supply purchasing capability. The New York City Department of Hospitals guarantees operation, maintenance, and administration of these municipal institutions, implying the continued availability of both nonprofessional personnel and funds. The affiliation approach appears in principle to be a straightforward redistribution of skilled physician power from affluent institutions to depleted ones. By this expedient, the city acknowledged its impotence to recruit and retain staff competent to deliver on an acceptable level the volume of services mandated by the City Charter. In entering upon an affiliation system, the city did not appear to consider the implications of separating the provision of professional services from routine hospital administration, of removing professional service provision from other than nominal public oversight, nor of giving the private institutions a direct voice in decision-making in essential government matters.

What were the factors that led to this profound imbalance in capability within the pluralistic system and the resultant paralysis of the public sector? Can the interest groups involved in fashioning this new policy be identified? Were there options that were overlooked or turned down by forces within government or the voluntary agencies? What have been the course and the accomplishments of the affiliation policy? Is it a viable and stable resolution of public-private hospital relationships?

Proponents of the policy contend that it is not essentially innovative, that it is an extension of the preexisting affiliative relationship between a segment of the hospital system and the local medical schools. Formally, this is true: major municipal hospitals had long been staffed by the universities, for example, Bellevue and Kings County, and decisions regarding the development and location of a new private medical school, Albert Einstein College of Medicine, were heavily influenced by the city's decision to build Bronx Municipal Hospital at its present site. These traditional arrangements provided access to patients for clinical instruction and experience for medical students under the supervision of the clinical staff selected, organized, and directed by the university from its own resources. The result of this *quid pro quo* was reputedly high-quality municipal service subsidized by private educational institutions. In addition to this structural connection, there has been an ongoing financial relationship between the city and the voluntary hospital system mediated by the city's charitable institutions' budget which reimburses non-city facilities on a uniform per diem basis for inpatient services to the indigent. In this sense the private sector has consistently supplemented the city's hospital care effort and, depending on the state of the general economy, this supplementation has been regarded either as a subsidy or as a financial drain.

The widely held belief that difficulties in staffing the municipal hospital system are distinctly a post-World War II phenomenon similarly requires qualification. Earlier surveys had also been concerned with the numerical inadequacy of annual medical school graduates to fill available house positions and the competitive disadvantage of smaller nonteaching hospitals in recruitment. In fact, municipal hospitals had long suffered other serious problems— failure of patients' confidence, public apathy, incompetence and indifference of visiting staff—which were determinants of the subsequent crisis in house staffing.

Hospital Department reports of the 1930s are illuminating. Dr. S. S. Goldwater, who was appointed to head the Department of Hospitals by Mayor LaGuardia at the beginning of his reform administration in 1934, found "the condition of the city's hospitals and institutions . . . so deplorable that to raise them to a desirable plane in the short space of a few years was impossible." The complaints of staff inadequacy, overcrowding, and insufficient appropriations resemble those of more recent investigations, though they derived from contemporary conditions: the depression, ubiquitous maladministration in municipal government, and the mandated dependence of municipal hospitals upon large numbers of uncompensated physicians for professional services in contradistinction to other city departments which paid the medical practitioners whom they employed. The Department of Hospitals was a substantial pork barrel, with staff administrative positions dispensed for political patronage and/or money. During the long depression of the 1930s, when eligibility for care at public expense characterized more than 60 percent of the population, municipal hospital admission rates resulted in patient loads in excess of 100 percent of capacity. As a consequence the city came to depend upon the voluntary system to treat the residual indigent load (some 30 percent of the total) by a combination of the voluntary system's own resources and per diem reimbursement. Municipal-voluntary hospital functioning in the prewar decade was characterized by excessive demand for free care with corresponding unsettling of both sectors: the public system strained its bed capacity while voluntary hospitals operated with incompletely utilized wards.

Structurally, during the thirties the municipal system underwent civil service reform, extension of the merit system, and more stringent regulation of purchasing and contract approvals, measures instituted to counteract political abuse. Control by the Director of the Budget, a position instituted in 1933 for sounder fiscal management, also had significant effects. Over time, these changes drastically attenuated the system's adaptability to postwar changing economic, technological, and labor market conditions. Throughout the two prewar decades the need of municipal institutions to cultivate closer relations with medical colleges and the need to approach standards of care analogous to those of liberally supported voluntary institutions reappear as policy themes. These preoccupations were reflective of a persistent trend to overvalue the privately administered institution in any situation where both private and public sectors were represented. Accordingly, affiliations between Kings County Hospital and Long Island College of Medicine and between Metropolitan Hospital and New York Medical College were negotiated in 1939.

A proposal to improve the city's capability to attract into its hospitals additional professional manpower by offering salaries for less than full-time service (surely an incentive during the depression) was only partially implemented; the City Charter was revised to permit a stipend for physicians serving in outpatient clinics on a session basis; visiting inpatient staff remained uncompensated.

During the postwar period, priority went to hospital construction to compensate for two decades of inactivity, first because of the depression, and later because of the military's requirements. The national commitment, concretized in the Hill-Burton legislation (1946), stimulated through generous matching funds extensive capital improvement in all hospital sectors. New York City, which had a low Hill-Burton priority relative to rural and less-developed urban areas, committed itself to a major construction program financed by a $150 million bond issue.

Plant maintenance, however, continued to be neglected so that serious obsolescence coexisted with new structures in the city's hospital plant. Conventional wisdom attributes the decline of the municipal hospitals to professional manpower depletion dating to the 1950s. Actually, for the nonteaching hospital, decline was a preexistent problem exacerbated by more generalized trends in medical care, some national in scale, others local. The chief determinants were technological: increasingly specialized, laboratory-oriented medical science, and hospital-based medical care, which in turn extended medical education from essentially undergraduate study with a terminal internship to formal postgraduate residency and specialty certification. Increased hospital demand, fairly fixed annual medical school output, and reduced internship period (from two years to one) directed almost all desirable house staff supply (i.e., graduates of American or Canadian medical schools) to teaching hospitals. This situation was a problem shared by both municipal and voluntary nonteaching hospitals. Government-stimulated clinical research further strengthened the recruitment power of the teaching hospital.

Economic changes, particularly in hospital care financing, also militated against the municipal institution. With increased hospital insurance coverage, there was an economic incentive in the form of admission privileges to the practitioner to serve the voluntary hospital, which in turn made increasing demands upon its staff. Between 1948 and 1958, an increase of between 15 to 20 percent occurred in municipal hospital appointments, but these were concentrated in university hospitals and in new hospitals; others suffered staff reduction. This increase contrasts poorly with an increase of 75 percent in voluntary hospitals. The greater attractiveness of staff appointments to voluntary hospitals is reflected in Klarman's finding that a majority of physicians who were municipal hospital attendings held dual appointments; only a minority of staff members of voluntary hospitals made this effort.

The decline of the municipal hospitals during the 1950s was neither precipitous nor mysterious, as it is frequently made out to be. It *was* shocking in the sense that by 1960 house staff attrition literally brought several facilities to the point of shutting down inpatient operations because of actual or threatened loss of accreditation; outpatient care was sporadic and disorganized, contingent from day to day upon the uncertain availability of attending physicians from the community. The municipal hospitals, even the most renowned, namely, Bellevue, had never been considered the equal of the great voluntary medical centers, New York Hospital, Presbyterian, or Mount Sinai, and by the late 1950s there were warnings, official and nonofficial, of generally substandard conditions and imminent collapse in specific units. To understand the factors behind this functional deterioration, a few fundamental distinctions should be made.

First, the critical inequality that developed in the hospital universe was not essentially between public and private hospitals, but between medical-school affiliated institutions and those nonaffiliated; this inequality determined their competitive positions with respect both to house staff recruitment and quality and continuity of attending staff. Medical school affiliation guaranteed attending staff of faculty rank in the municipal hospital; such a guarantee, in turn, was a magnet for drawing American-educated interns and residents, perhaps in somewhat smaller numbers than the prestigious voluntary hospitals but nonetheless adequate.

Severe underfinancing, obsolescence and plant deterioration, and bureaucratic management have been cited as causes of the loss of operating capability of the municipal system. These were chronic problems which became actually disabling when radical technological and structural changes in medicine took place during the post-World War II years (1945–60). These changes were reflected in an altered production function, altered training structure, altered relations among providers of services. Increasing orders of specialization and subspecialization and an expanding substratum of laboratory tests and procedures for diagnosis and therapy shifted the medical center of gravity irrevocably to the hospital, specifically the hospital closest to the scientific source, that is, the medical school or teaching hospital.

The development of specialized medicine led simultaneously to the institution of formal training structures requisite for specialty certification, again centered in the medical school with its concentration of scientific facilities and personnel. The leading voluntary hospitals, with greater access to funds and with more administrative freedom, adapted readily to both physical requirements and the need for changed staffing patterns and mixes. Full-time chiefs of staff were introduced into twelve nonaffiliated hospitals, most of them Jewish, as the inadequacies of attendings in the changed production function became apparent, and salaries and fringe benefits were made competitive with income from private practice. Part-time employment followed, with the net effect of drawing off the best of the teacher clinicians, particularly younger men who received their graduate medical training in the postwar years.

What staff remained in the unaffiliated municipal institutions was a diminishing number of older clinicians. Although most of these hospitals were officially accredited for a variety of specialty residences, they were the boondocks of the educational structure and hospital practice failed to attract American-trained medical graduates. Accordingly, house staff once attracted to the municipal hospitals which offered rich general medical and surgical experience, invaluable for the broad-based general practice of pre-World War II, now were drawn to hospitals providing differential training for the highly specialized practice that has predominated since. The federal largess in underwriting specialty training for military medical personnel and veterans reinforced an already irresistible trend and further unbalanced the distribution of physician manpower between the public and private hospital sectors.

The difficulties wrought by the failure of the city hospitals to adapt adequately to new medical techniques were compounded by serious postwar demographic shifts. Changes in population distribution, that is, the outflow of the white middle class from older residential areas in the city to new communities on the periphery or in the suburbs, and their replacement in town by in-migrating blacks and Puerto Ricans, impoverished populations, left most of the municipal hospitals in deteriorating neighborhoods with a rapidly aging, dwindling physician population, unreplenished by younger men. With no local private practice, physicians providing services at the public hospital, previously offered partly as community service, partly for local prestige, partly because the hospital was utilized by their marginal patients, suffered attrition. Others relocated. Drainage of the middle class drained physicians' services simultaneously.

With the increasing enrollment of hospital insurance plans, the municipal hospitals, which had traditionally served the medically indigent (a loosely defined group which included much of the lower-income employed population who received ambulatory services from local private practitioners), lost this population to the voluntary hospitals, and with them much of the municipal hospitals' claim on the professional services of the local physicians. Public hospitals became a resource, on both an inpatient and an outpatient level, primarily for the very poor who were outside the structure of private medicine. At the nonteaching level, the public hospitals constituted an institutional affiliation only for older loyal staff members and a heterogeneous set of physicians who were employed on a fractional time basis, the "sessions" men.

The extent of municipal hospital deterioration was publicized through two communications, one from a group of department heads of Columbia University's College of Physicians and Surgeons at Bellevue (1957) and the other from a city-wide committee of interns and residents of municipal hospitals (1958–59). These early warnings were followed by two formal studies, one by the *ad hoc* Commission on Health Services in the City of New York (Heyman Commission), another by the Hospital Council of Greater New York (*New York City and Its Hospitals*), each of which was reported in 1960. Both studies found widespread deterioration in municipal hospital operations owing to the interplay of underfinancing and understaffing and chaotic and dangerous conditions at isolated facilities. The elimination of the latter was recommended through two actions: closing obsolete facilities and integrating units containing viable plants with major teaching institutions. Despite a clear difference in focus between the Heyman Commission, which addressed itself to the spectrum of public health services, and the Hospital Council's concern with municipal-voluntary relations, both studies proceeded on the assumption that quality medical care depends on intimate links with teaching and research. Both looked to the medical school as the center in the organization and provision of community health care, a position far from universally accepted by the medical academic community, much less by the active practitioner. The Heyman report explicitly committed itself to the principle of medical-school-centered regionalization of medical care.

Actual implementation of the hospital affiliation system was effected, however, as an emergency measure following the loss of accreditation by Gouverneur Hospital, of specific residency programs at Greenpoint and other hospitals, and the disqualification of most of the house staff at Harlem Hospital because of their failure to pass a mandatory foreign graduates' examination instituted in 1961. Dr. Ray Trussell, on leave from Columbia University, was appointed Commissioner of Hospitals by Mayor Robert Wagner with a promise of unqualified support. Trussell's administration, which was extended to 1965, succeeded in contracting out professional services for all city institutions but for two anomalies, Sydenham and Seaview.

What have been the chief characteristics of these affiliations? The most conspicuous aspect of Trussell's policy was its *ad hoc* character. Individual contracts varied considerably in scope and value. The affiliations ranged from limited interdepartmental relationships between Harlem Hospital and the College of Physicians and Surgeons to complete responsibility by the affiliate for all professional and auxiliary operations (Montefiore-Morrisania). Beth Israel assumed responsibility for comprehensive ambulatory services at Gouverneur, following closure of the inpatient services.

The affiliations were not implemented systematically. They were negotiated for an initial term of three years on an individual basis, the most urgent situations first, the least critical (hence the most likely to be opposed) last. Common to all the affiliations was the responsibility of the voluntary hospital to provide professional (i.e., medical) services including supervision of the house staff. Full-time chiefships were written into each contract; it was assumed that quality house staff recruitment, hitherto unsuccessful, would thereby be facilitated. The city retained responsibility for hospital administration, plant maintenance, and provision of supplies and supportive personnel. Reimbursement to the affiliate was on a cost-plus-overhead (10 percent) basis. The first contract round was characterized by few constraints, liberal terms, limited fiscal auditing, and an absence of quality auditing of hospital services. Contract renewals at the expiration of the initial three-year period were generally marked by enlargement of scope, greater contract uniformity, and clear city surveillance.

In the crisis atmosphere of initial contract negotiation in 1961, monetary constraints were loosened, if not abandoned altogether. Principally, contracting was adopted as a means of circumventing the city's line-item budgeting in the reorganization of municipal staffs, and of release from the anachronistic salary structure of civil service, permitting expenditures "according to the prevailing practices of the affiliating institution." Additionally, the affiliate was given some freedom for emergency purchase of supplies and equipment. With *ad hoc* contract negotiation to meet emergencies, costs were not seriously considered; there were no budgeting guidelines, no uniformity of record maintenance, and infrequent fiscal auditing. Contracts were defended individually before the Board of Estimate by Trussell, who initially estimated a cost of "a few million dollars or so" to the city. The actual budgets of the contracts have risen steadily to become a sizeable proportion of the total Hospital Department's expenditure. Since 1967 the contracts have approximated one-third of the Department's budget.

Year	Contract value (in millions)
1961	$ 3
1966	84
1967	121
1969–70	137

These escalating sums reflect the increasing number of hospitals that have been included within the affiliation network and, more significantly, the increasing scope of services, medical and ancillary, for which affiliates have assumed responsibility. Inflationary hospital employment costs, propelled in part by the freer bargaining practices of the voluntary network, have been a significant factor. The inclusion under contract of institutions serving the direct teaching needs of the medical schools, for example, Metropolitan and Bellevue (1967), which had formerly assumed staffing costs themselves, has accounted for substantial increases.

In addition to more stringent auditing requirements, closer regulation of professional practices, and some restrictions on allowable ancillary expenses, the chief direct efforts to limit the encroachment of affiliation costs on the Hospital Department budget have been freezing job transfers (for nonprofessional categories) from civil service to contract payrolls at 1967 levels, and cutting back affiliation overhead allowances from an over-all 10 percent of costs to a declining percentage contingent on the value of the contract, with a minimum of 5 percent for amounts in excess of $4 million.

A look at affiliations reveals benefits not only to the recipients but to the providers of services. The strongest and most heavily committed are Einstein, Mount Sinai, Montefiore, Maimonides, and Beth Israel, aggressive institutions, committed to the medical-school teaching-research-centered model of health service leadership and organization, underendowed in terms of their expanding educational and research programs and staff. With the growth of insurance, affiliation offered them a substantial increase of service (teaching) beds and ambulatory patients to supplement their shrinking supply, and additional funds with which to obtain quality staff in an expensive market. To the weaker institutions, for example, Misericordia and Mary Immaculate, it offered the possibility of financial strengthening and professional upgrading to the level of teaching hospitals rather than permanent retreat to the ranks of mediocre community hospitals and the disaccreditation of existing residencies. Middle-rank teaching hospitals, such as Brooklyn Jewish and Brooklyn, also anticipated financial bolstering and improved status. The blue chips of the medical school universe, with substantial funds of their own or from the federal government without encumbrances, and having an exclusionary view of public responsibility, either refused to participate (Cornell–New York Hospital) or undertook limited programs (Columbia–Presbyterian Hospital).

In building bridges between the academic medical and clinical teaching complex and the municipal hospitals for the restoration of acceptable professional services in the hospitals through the extension of their own abundant manpower resources, which Commissioner Trussell saw as the primary objective of his administration, he avoided any analogous approach to administrative services. In contrast to limited clinician personnel, hospital administrative officers, physician-careerists in the civil service, were very much present in the individual municipal facilities and resented, and in several cases bitterly opposed, the replacement of their own clinical appointees and the usurpation of their powers of staff appointment and dismissal by the respective chiefs of service of the affiliating hospital. The hospital administrators and internal management structures that Trussell inherited covered the range of weak to powerful.

In theory, professional policy in a municipal hospital is established by the Medical Board and is independent of the administrator, whose influence and functions are limited to specific areas. On the other hand, a strong hospital administrator may control the Medical Board. In the municipal system, he is also responsible for negotiations with allocative, purchasing, personnel, and policy-determining agencies within the central bureaucracy. As in the case of professional personnel, the inefficient, frustrating, and underfinanced city administrative function combined with an anachronistic salary schedule had permitted an outflow of managerial skill during the 1940s and 1950s, leaving the system with a few powerful superintendents, well connected politically, who managed their institutions like independent fiefdoms, and a larger number of mediocre executives. A few amenable superintendents undertook the administrative responsibilities of the affiliation, but by and large harmonious integration of city and affiliate services did not occur. External liaison and internal management problems were mediated centrally within the Commissioner's office and minimal effective authority was retained by the local hospital administrator. As a result, there was a residue of internal dissension, divided operations, and failure of coordination among the city, the affiliate professional staff, and the local administration.

Prepotence of the affiliate was further augmented by the easy transfer of individual jobs from civil service to contract, as employees either left or were terminated. The trend toward increased administrative centralization and the erosion of local civil service employment and authority persisted throughout Trussell's administration and the brief term of his successor, Alonzo Yerby. The growing restiveness of the city officialdom and of District Council No. 37 of the American Federation of State, County, and Municipal Employees (headed by Victor Gotbaum) culminated in the major investigations of 1966—an intensive fiscal audit by City Comptroller Mario Procaccino and an operations review by the New York State Blue Ribbon Panel—which served as the first watershed in the course of the affiliation system.

The more heavily publicized findings of these investigations revolved about evidence of injudicious expenditures for office and research equipment and nonpatient care activities, diversion of physician time from direct medical services to research and teaching, loose timekeeping and bookkeeping. Nevertheless, at least three basic problem areas emerged: divided management, inadequate departmental supervision (professional), and the persistent failure of the city to meet its contractual functions—maintenance of the hospital plant, supply, purchase, and housekeeping, supportive and security services. As a result, under Commissioner Joseph Terenzio, there was a distinct shift of departmental focus in the direction of developing an effectively decentralized managerial structure and limiting the expanding authority of the affiliates.

From an *ad hoc* heterogeneous set of municipal-voluntary contractual relationships that could be considered a system only in terms of the objectives and executive practice of Dr. Trussell, there emerged under the administration of Commissioner Terenzio greater uniformity of mutual obligations and, more importantly, a rationalized administrative model with clearer definition of local and central administrative function.

Commissioner Terenzio was the first nonmedical man to head the Hospitals Department. Yerby, like Trussell, was a physician, a public health careerist, with a liberal medical-school orientation and predominantly programmatic and quality concerns; Terenzio, on the other hand, is a hospital administrator. One of his first moves was in the direction of decentralizing the affiliation network, which in its early years had spun rather unevenly around the Commissioner as prime mover. An unmitigated source of difficulty in municipal-voluntary relations had been the impotence of the individual city hospital directors in dealing with the innumerable officials in the city bureaucracy whom it was necessary to consult on all but the most insignificant aspects of hospital management. Every study of the municipal hospital system, beginning with the Report of the Mayor's Commission on Health Services (Heyman Commission, 1960), has drawn attention to the strangling effect upon hospital management of the city's redoubtable regulatory apparatus governing all aspects of personnel (hiring and firing) and financial expenditures. It is no surprise, therefore, that imaginative managerial talent has not been drawn to the system. Further deterrence came from the low salary scale and from the requirement that only a physician could qualify for the position of hospital director. The affiliation contracts stripped the hospital administrator of his former effective power by removing his authority over professional staff and services.

With respect to affiliation contracts, coordination, the establishment of general policy and operating guidelines, contract interpretation, and fiscal oversight were lodged in 1967 in an Office of Affiliations directed by an administrator at the assistant commissioner level. In a series of directives this office introduced limitations and regulations governing such matters as timekeeping, purchase, payroll, and standards. Contracts were similarly redrawn for greater specificity and uniformity, and a unit value of equating services was devised as a basis for budgetary computation. Job transfers over a wide range of aides and nontechnical categories from city to affiliate payroll were frozen as of early 1967. The direction of the recent administration was to fix more firmly the inherent dualism of the system: professional services deriving from the voluntary sector with its distinctive standards and interests, and management devolving upon the city with a separate set of constraints and commitments. In the area of program review, where such differences of commitment and outlook might be mediated, the Affiliations Office accomplished little.

With the commencement of operations by the New York City Health and Hospitals Corporation in July, 1970, the Affiliations Office was absorbed by the new structure and continued its functions under a slightly altered title, Office of Affiliation Administration, with its director, the former deputy assistant commissioner, renamed executive assistant and responsible to the Corporation director. For the first year at least, affiliation contracts and operations will continue essentially unchanged.

In the wake of the City Comptroller's audits of the Hospitals Department, a Commission on the Delivery of Personal Health Services, consisting of seven citizen members, representative of neither professional nor technical health interests, under the chairmanship of Gerard Piel, was appointed by Mayor John Lindsay in December, 1966, "to make a thorough inquiry into the institutional, administrative and fiscal aspects of the system through which public funds now deliver personal health services to one-third of the people of New York City" and to make specific recommendations for implementation by the Health Services Administration. Closely allied to the Commission were two physicians, co-chairmen of a Medical Advisory Committee for guidance in professional and medical aspects of the study, and its staff director, a nonphysician administrator. Funded generously by private foundations, the Commission was enabled to extend its investigations with exhaustive studies by a field staff, whose published findings (1969) supplement and document the official Commission Report (December, 1967).

The report reveals a shift in focus from the Commission's original, more narrowly conceived mandate respecting publicly funded services to a wider interpretation of the city's total health commitment to its citizenry, encompassing the entire health services system. The title of the report is *Comprehensive Community Health Services for New York City*. Beyond its basic findings that compromised hospital services are inevitable under the obsolescent conditions of the municipal hospital plant, and that ambulatory care and long-term care are tragically inadequate, the report was fundamentally critical of the dual system of public (welfare) and private medicine. The basic thrust of its recommendation was toward an idealistic coordination and integration of both systems into a regional model under the authority of the city. Specifically recommended were: (1) the coordination of all city health agencies under a single Health Services Administration with planning, monitoring, standard-setting, inspection, review, and coordinating functions (its designation by the State of New York to organize the federally funded comprehensive health-planning agency, under Public Law 79-849, was strongly urged); (2) creation of a nonprofit health services corporation to integrate the current institutional network within a single, decentralized, comprehensive regional system. The corporation was to assume operation of the city's existing health centers and facilities and responsibility for plant maintenance and rehabilitation; additionally it was empowered to construct health facilities to be operated by itself or by voluntary agencies. Significantly, the Commission counseled against autonomous financing of the corporation's capital and operating requirements, among other reasons to maintain city control over the system.

By mid-1969 two recommendations of the Commission had been adopted. After a long struggle with the Health and Hospital Planning Council of Southern New York, the thirty-year-old nonprofit planning organization that was heavily reflective of the voluntary health care system, the Health Services Administration, instituted in 1967 to integrate the four major municipal health agencies, was designated to organize the Comprehensive Health Planning Agency. In addition, the state legislature enacted the New York City Health and Hospitals Corporation Act, a considerably modified version of the original Piel Commission proposal.

How did reality differ from the ideal? Basically, the New York City Health and Hospitals Corporation is an instrument aimed at overcoming the most egregious deficiencies of capital construction and operation of municipal health facilities by circumventing the city's rigid budgeting and personnel practices, the interminable construction process, and the extreme administrative centralization. A key facet is that the Corporation has no responsibility for non-public facilities. The main thrust of the Piel Report—to replace the traditional parallelism with a single, publicly accountable, decentralized health care system—was clearly ahead of its time, and those specific proposals which were unacceptable to the entrenched interest groups who control the major components of the system—institutions, money, manpower—were subjected to negotiations that eventuated in the revised Corporation. Specifically:

1. The voluntary institutions, unprepared to cede control to an authority wholly appointed by the city and accountable to the city, were omitted from the Corporation.

2. The unions, representing both public employees (District Council No. 37, American Federation of State, County, and Municipal Employees) and private employees (Local 1199, Drug and Hospital Employees Union), were unwilling to relinquish their control. Hence the community control proposals were modified. An indefinite future commitment was embodied in the Corporation's authority to form and contract with local subcorporations.

Except in the case of Harlem Hospital, no action could be taken for at least two years, and any future subcorporation is explicitly restricted from altering city-determined personnel policies and from engaging in collective bargaining or union negotiations. The Corporation is legally bound to protect civil service employment and collective bargaining agreements.

3. The city, unwilling to lose its title to public institutions or to abandon fiscal control, has restricted the Corporation's right to issue construction bonds without the agreement of the mayor and to dispose of property without the consent of the Board of Estimate. More importantly, the city is also the source for supplemental and deficit funding, thereby retaining—via the Bureau of the Budget, as in the past—fiscal control over operations. Five of the sixteen members of the board of directors are mandated city officials, any four of whom hold veto power over majority decisions.

4. The politicians, unprepared to withdraw from participating in a municipal service offering public exposure and patronage potential, reserved for the City Council the right to designate one-third of the directors.

In brief, the Corporation extends and broadens the principle underlying affiliation contracts. Its functions encompass both construction and operation, provide greater public accountability and cost control, and coordinate administration and service under one umbrella. The anticipated effect of this new instrumentality will be to enhance municipal services in any single area where the urgent plight of the system is acknowledged by all health interests. But it is not likely to result in any essential change in the present dual system of hospital care.

In light of the politically motivated municipal (Procaccino) and state (Lane Commission) investigations of the hospital affiliations and the more considered and objective studies of the Piel Commission and the Burney Commission (Blue Ribbon Panel to Governor Nelson A. Rockefeller on Municipal Hospitals of New York City, Report, 1967), it is reasonable to ask what has actually been the outcome of this bold intervention into the ongoing municipal hospital function. From the evidence, a fair answer would be that the contracts have delivered the agreed-to services, namely, to staff the city institutions with competent professional manpower, and to appoint full-time senior men to direct the individual departments under the supervision of the corresponding director in the affiliate hospital, thereby strengthening the professional aspects of patient care. The ancillary services included in the contracts have similiarly been improved, although these vary with the strength of the affiliate. The modest decentralization written into the contracts has demonstrated the potentialities of freeing the system from the bureaucratic rigidities and fiscal constraints of municipal operation. While the hospitals have not been made over (a 1969 reportorial survey by the New York *Times* revealed the persistence of the by now familiar decrepitude and inadequacy of most of the facilities), procurement of some essential supplies and equipment has been expedited by direct purchase.

The cost to the city has risen annually, amounting in the 1969–70 executive budget to approximately $140 million, 15 percent of a total health budget of about $1 billion. At this level of expenditure, the question arises whether there has been a commensurate yield to the city. Certainly there is a similarity (more than a suggestion of resemblance) to the inflationary effect of the large-scale federally subsidized programs. With monies of this magnitude dispensed on a program basis, the city might well exercise program control by a greater degree of specificity and standard-setting in the contracts and by regular program audits and reviews. Thus far, government investigations have focused upon fiscal irresponsibility, waste, and misappropriation in place of the improvement of services to the poor that was the program's primary intent. The disclosures have resulted in tighter budgetary control and a partial regression in the direction of line-item specification, from the original program approach that Dr. Trussell instituted with the first set of contracts. Under the Corporation it should be possible finally to maintain fiscal accountability and review of the affiliation program without recourse to line budgeting, which the affiliation system was designed to avoid.

The affiliations have greatly increased the influence of the voluntary sector upon municipal medical service; the powerful voluntary "establishment," which formerly exercised indirect veto powers in municipal decision-making, has had a greatly strengthened voice, at least within the Hospitals Department. The city has failed to develop any comparable degree of control over the voluntary sector in terms of goals and objectives, program evaluation, and standard-setting. If the value of the contracts is augmented by the Charitable Institutions Budget, which is currently of the order of $125 million (payment for inpatient care, *exclusive* of professional services and of ambulatory services for Medicaid eligibles and non-Medicaid indigent), the minimum subvention to the voluntary hospitals exceeds $300 million, over which the city exercises little effective control.

An implicit assumption behind much of the controversy over the limited accomplishment of the affiliation system has been that the contracts should serve as a first step toward equalization of the parallel hospital systems by the extension to the municipal facilities of university standards and objectives (Piel Report), an expectation that was reinforced with the introduction of Medicaid. The illusoriness of this assumption has been reflected in the decreased utilization of the municipal hospitals under conditions of substantial consumer-choice, namely (pre-cutback) Medicaid and Medicare. A more judicious assessment might be that the affiliation experience has brought the two systems into closer relationship, primarily at the level of younger staff. However, this relationship has raised some basic questions: whether the university hospital is an apposite model and whether the university hospital type of service should be generally extended to the poor for whose care the city is responsible. There has been some experimentation with differential services and differential organization at some centers to meet specific needs of the local principal hospital constituency, but there has been no explicit consideration of these factors by the city in the course of reaching its contractual agreements with the affiliate hospital. Another, somewhat allied effect results from the fact that there are now attending physicians in various hospitals who have been alienated through replacement or reduction in status and to whom the community has turned, particularly under Medicaid and Medicare, for nonhospital care. The nonhospital-affiliated physician, with marginal professional ability, is an additional wedge between the community and more effective medical service, toward which affiliation was a proposed instrument.

If we were to recapitulate the course and outcome of the affiliation system in the perspective of a reasonable operational period (almost one decade), we would see it as an innovative response negotiated for the city by an outside professional, Commissioner Trussell, to cope with the chronic problem of understaffing that had reached a critical stage, and that was deteriorating at an exponential rate, with politically explosive consequences. Although the affiliation system involved the concentration of considerable power by its proponent, a nonpolitician, it offered a politically attractive solution—the promise of reviving and revitalizing the municipal system at apparently little cost by the expedient of redistributing the superior professional manpower of the competitor voluntary system. Essentially, the municipal hospitals would be transfused back to institutional health. But what was the definition of institutional health?

Over time, the dual system has developed two distinct, if overlapping, sets of assumptions regarding objectives against which quality must be assayed. Municipal hospitals are committed to provide medical services to the poor; the objectives of the voluntary sector, specifically its most exemplary subset, the teaching hospitals, are explicitly multifunctional—patient care, clinical instruction, and research constitute an interlocking triad which informs both policy and standards. In contracting with the teaching hospitals for service *implicitly* at their level of quality, the city gave little hard thought to the cost and functional implications of such an alliance. The innovative relationship in the fluid hospital system did not simply fill a void; it developed a momentum of its own with unanticipated consequences for both networks. The claim of the voluntary institutions upon city financing was extended beyond historic tax abatement and per diem reimbursement for care of indigent patients, to payment for the application of their standards of professional service in the operation of the municipal hospitals. With the outreach of this new standard it became increasingly evident with the passage of time that the infusion of physician manpower alone into the municipal system would not suffice to ensure quality care in the face of inadequacies in allied professional services—nursing, clinical technology, social service—which were more difficult to remedy because of steeply rising wages throughout the entire system. In addition, during the decade of the 1960s in-hospital appointments (internships and residencies which constituted the bulk of the staffing) were transformed from inexpensive to increasingly expensive service and salaried supervisory personnel replaced the previously available free visiting staff. Consequently, the cost of the contracts grew to a level substantially different from Trussell's original estimate. The availability of Medicare-Medicaid funds beginning in 1966 enabled the city to meet the open-ended costs of affiliation and postponed the inevitable reconsideration of a program that aimed to provide improved services for the poor under the existent institutional arrangements.

What was the nature of the city's plan to upgrade its hospitals? Essentially, the affiliation contracts constitute a system of inputs linked to a conceptualized but undefined output, "quality care." Given the unresolved problems of quality and output measurement inherent in the production of medical services and the affiliation system's passivity even in the areas of program review and overview, what could eventuate? Despite avowed improvement, grave systemic deficiencies persist—deficiencies that are discernible to any observer and that have been repeatedly documented by investigation.

With increasing expenditure of public funds, there has been a reversion to the classic strategy of meeting public criticism and the exposure of deficiencies with the imposition of administrative restrictions and an at least partial return to the *status quo ante* of tight fiscal control. This sequence is inevitable in the area of tax-funded services.

A more definitive strategy for the enhancement of municipal health services in light of the affiliations might be to consider more directly the output of quality service. If the present posture of the city is to continue, that is, if it is to provide services for the poor (increasing numbers of whom are eligible for third-party nonmunicipal reimbursement) through its own apparatus, and not to infringe directly, if at all, on the autonomy of the voluntary system, how can it maximize the yield from its resources? Could monies be transferred to the voluntary institutions to provide defined care, perhaps on a per capita basis, to a defined population in order to alleviate the extremes of distributive inequity? What institutional changes can be effected to reduce inefficiency? Would it be feasible for the city hospitals to be reorganized into a supplemental, rather than a parallel, system vis-à-vis the voluntary hospitals, effecting a true functional differentiation in the services that the two networks provide? For instance, might they transfer patients requiring highly specialized care? Would it be feasible to make available beds for private patients in city as well as voluntary institutions?

The affiliation experience has been, in a sense, analogous to the Medicare-Medicaid experience: the extension of additional resources to the poor and to the institutions serving the poor has not equalized the services available in a complex, unequal system. Perhaps the lesson of these large-scale reform efforts should be the bold and unequivocal recognition that a dual system precludes equality. In that case, policy and program formulation must be directed at rationalization of function and structure in the two systems in order to optimize a defined output rather than to pursue an illusory, if time-honored, objective.

6

EMERGENCY ROOM SERVICES

SINCE THE BEGINNING of the 1960s visits to hospital emergency rooms in New York City have increased at a rate far exceeding the rates of increase in the use of other hospital facilities. This chapter will describe the trends in emergency room use and seek to explain them. It will suggest that the hospitals responded to the increased demand for emergency room care by means of *ad hoc* adaptations rather than by planning.

A properly planned and staffed emergency room—as distinguished from a clinic—should be able to care for a child with a broken arm, for the victim of an automobile accident, for an elderly patient with a heart attack, as well as for the minor aches and pains which often propel a patient to seek care. Many emergency rooms, however, do not seem able to accomplish these multiple tasks, either because of inadequate technical facilities or because of insufficient staff.

TRENDS

The total number of visits to emergency rooms per year grew from approximately 1.8 million in 1960 to over 2.7 million in 1967, representing an acceleration of an earlier trend. The rate of growth in emergency room visits far exceeded the rate of increase recorded for outpatient departments or inpatient days, as Table 6.1 demonstrates.

In fact, outpatient visits, which climbed steadily until 1965, *declined* from 1965 to 1967, while the number of inpatient days showed only a modest increase throughout the period 1961 to 1967.

TABLE 6.1

Utilization of Hospital Services in New York City, 1961–1967

(in millions)

Type of Service and Type of Hospital	1961	1962	1963	1964	1965	1966	1967
Emergency room visits—total	1.98	2.16	2.31	2.50	2.66	2.64	2.73
Municipal hospitals	1.14	1.27	1.39	1.53	1.62	1.51	1.47
Voluntary hospitals	.84	.89	.92	.97	1.04	1.13	1.26
Outpatient department visits—total	5.72	5.79	5.88	6.11	6.26	6.15	5.89
Municipal hospitals	2.79	2.80	2.90	3.09	3.28	3.39	3.11
Voluntary hospitals	2.93	2.99	2.98	3.02	2.98	2.76	2.78
Inpatient days—total	n.a.	10.74	10.65	10.94	10.96	11.10	11.41
Municipal hospitals	n.a.	2.88	2.81	2.74	2.75	2.69	2.64
Voluntary hospitals	n.a.	6.56	6.67	6.87	6.98	7.10	7.35
Proprietary hospitals	n.a.	1.30	1.17	1.33	1.23	1.31	1.42

Sources: Emergency room visits—United Hospital Fund mimeographed report.
Outpatient department visits and inpatient days—New York City Department of Hospitals, Annual Report, 1967.
n.a. = Not available. However, The Health and Hospitals Corporation reports a total figure for all sectors of 10.5 million.

Emergency room visits, by contrast, show a marked and steady rise in volume, since they offered perhaps the only alternative, particularly for the poor, to secure medical attention in the face of a shrinking supply of family physicians practicing in slum areas.

Until 1965 the municipal hospitals accounted for a disproportionate share of the demand for emergency room care: during the 1960-65 period their rate of increase was about twice that of the voluntary hospitals. But between 1965 and 1967 a definite shift occurred. Table 6.1 shows that in those years annual emergency room visits to voluntary hospitals increased from 1.04 to 1.26 million, while visits to municipal hospitals declined from 1.62 to 1.47 million.

In addition to the increased use of emergency rooms and the shift from municipal to voluntary hospitals, a third trend appeared: a change in type of patient served, reflecting the changing demographic character of New York City.

National studies of emergency room populations in urban settings have revealed: (1) more children and young adults; (2) more males; (3) more nonmarried patients; (4) more nonwhite clients; (5) more inner-city residents; (6) more persons of lower socioeconomic status; (7) more people of limited education; (8) more people from low-income neighborhoods; (9) more people without a regular relationship to a personal physician; and (10) more persons from households where the head is unemployed.[1]

CHANGING FUNCTION OF THE
EMERGENCY ROOM

In recent years, while the number of emergency room visits has increased signicantly, a marked change has occurred in the nature of patient services. The most significant have been: (1) the disproportionate increase in the number of patients with nonemergency problems; (2) the dependence on the urban hospital by the medically indigent in the "core city."

Recent studies show that most patients demanding emergency room services do not need immediate attention but still seek it. According to the National Research Council, over two-thirds of all emergency room visits in 1966 could not be classified as emergencies.[2] The emergency rooms of hospitals that have been studied appear to serve different populations, treat different medical complaints, and treat them differently.

One of the most important differences found among emergency rooms is the relationship between the hospital and private practitioners. At hospitals located in higher-income areas, the number of patients who have a private physician is much higher than in low-income areas; these patients use the emergency room only as a supplement to seeking services from their physician. In low-income areas, the emergency room substitutes for the private physician. A 1965 study of four New York City hospitals showed that emergency rooms located in middle- and high-income areas treat patients who, facing an emergency and unable to make contact with their regular physician, seek stopgap help.[3] Normally, these people obtain their medical care in their physician's office and use the emergency room as a backup.

By contrast, the lower-income patients using emergency rooms do not have private physicians, and look to the emergency room as their basic source of medical attention. They view the emergency room not merely as a place to obtain treatment for minor illness but as an entree, when needed, to the hospital's more intricate services. Thus, the emergency room has become, in the absence of any effective alternative, the primary source of medical care for a significant portion of New York City's population.

If the average number of emergency room visits per patient were known, an estimate of the city's population that relies upon the emergency room for their primary medical care could be made. Even in the absence of such information, an estimate can be ventured. For example, in 1967 there were a total of 2.73 million emergency room visits. If one postulates an average number of visits per patient of between two and six, emergency rooms were providing primary medical care for a minimum of 450,000 persons (six visits per person) to a high of 1.4 million, if we assume two visits per patient.

Interviews of 1,113 emergency room patients, conducted in the 1965 study of four New York hospitals, revealed that approximately

30 percent of all doctor-patient contacts among this population made in the previous year occurred in the emergency room. This figure varied significantly, from almost 40 percent for one hospital located in a low-income area to approximately 20 percent for another in a middle-income area.[4] One probable cause for the great increase in use of the emergency room is the decreasing availability of private general practitioners, particularly in low-income areas of the city.

The number of general practitioners has decreased throughout the city primarily because more physicians now specialize. Those remaining in general practice no longer make themselves readily available for house calls; instead, they often refer patients to emergency rooms. In addition, they frequently arrange to meet their patients in the emergency room of the hospital, where diagnostic facilities and supportive personnel are readily available. Over 10 percent of the patients interviewed in a 1965 study of New York Hospital had been directed to the emergency room by their own physicians.[5]

The problem of physician shortage is exacerbated in ghettos: there are a declining number of private practitioners; those who retire or die are often not replaced; and even when a general practitioner continues to maintain his office in the ghetto, the poor cannot afford to use him. In the Gouverneur Medical Service Area, a low-income area in lower Manhattan, the number of private physicians declined from 158 in 1963 to 109 in 1967—a drop of 31 percent in four years.[6]

FINANCING

The expanded use of emergency rooms may be partly explained by the changing patterns of financing medical care. The increase in the availability of third-party reimbursement for emergency room visits played a significant role in the expansion of emergency room services and in the shift of patients from municipal to voluntary hospital emergency rooms, in particular after the introduction of Medicaid.

Blue Cross policies have also contributed to the rise in emergency room use. Blue Cross includes a cash allowance for emergency outpatient care, that is, emergency room care, received within twenty-four hours after a person has suffered an accidental injury. However, this coverage affects only a minor fraction of all emergency room services and an infinitesimal portion of those provided in the municipal hospitals. In New York City during 1967, for example, 254,497 visits were reimbursed (less than 10 percent of a total of 2.7 million), 98.5 percent to voluntary and proprietary hospitals, 1.5 percent to municipal hospitals. The total reimbursement amounted to $2.8 million, almost all of which went to voluntary and proprietary hospitals, in partial payment of charges averaging $19.79 and $18.07 respectively. Because its plans do not cover visits to private physicians, Blue Cross has been indirectly encouraging subscribers to seek medical care in emergency rooms, where the patient's emergency expenditures are reimbursed.

However, not everyone has Blue Cross coverage. In fact, the Torrens study revealed a striking difference between the percentage of insured patients in hospitals in middle- and upper-income areas in contrast to those in hospitals in lower-income areas. Among the hospitals from which our data were gathered, the percentage with insurance ranged from 80 percent in high-income areas to 30 percent in one ghetto hospital.

The Medicaid enrollment campaign took place during 1966. Therefore we must look at patterns of hospital use from 1965 through 1967 to understand the effects of Medicaid. The number of visits shows a definite shift in the pattern of utilization of emergency rooms in New York City. In voluntary hospitals an 8.2 percent increase occurred in 1966 followed by a further 11.5 percent increase in 1967, compared to average annual increases of only 5.3 percent during the 1961-65 period. The municipal hospitals, on the other hand, experienced a 6.8 percent decrease in 1966, followed by a further 3.3 percent decrease in 1967. These declines contrast with average annual increases of 8.6 percent during the 1961-65 period (see Table 6.2).

In 1967 the Department of Social Services, which administers Medicaid in New York City, paid $10.1 million to private physicians for services rendered to ambulatory Medicaid patients. This sum represented 41 percent of the total payment ($24.5 million)

TABLE 6.2

Visits to Emergency Rooms of New York City Hospitals, 1965–1967

	Percent of Average Annual Increase 1961–65	1965 Number of Visits	1966 Number of Visits	Percent of Change 1965–66	1967 Number of Visits	Percent of Change 1966–67
Voluntary hospitals	+5.3	1,040,682	1,125,667	+8.2	1,255,090	+11.5
Municipal hospitals	+8.6	1,624,128	1,514,724	−6.8	1,465,603	− 3.3
Total		2,664,810	2,640,391	−3.0	2,720,693	+ 3.0

Source: United Hospital Fund.

made by the Department for such patients during that year.[7] Over $12 million, or 49 percent, was paid to voluntary hospitals for outpatient department and emergency room services, while only $2.3 million, or 9.3 percent, was paid for emergency room services in the municipal hospital system. Thus the effect of Medicaid was to funnel funds to private physicians and voluntary hospitals, with only small sums going to municipal hospitals. These shifts reflect latent dissatisfaction of many poor people with the quality of emergency room care in municipal hospitals.

It is also of interest to compare the payments made by the Welfare Department in 1965 to private physicians, voluntary hospitals, and municipal hospitals under its several public assistance programs with the payments for ambulatory services covered by Medicaid which were reimbursed by the Department of Social Services during 1967. The increase in total money flows between 1965 and 1967 was more than ninefold, from $2.7 million to $24.5 million. The payments to private physicians showed the greatest increase—from less than $275,000 to over $10 million (an increase of about forty times). The payments to voluntary hospitals increased about seven times, from $1.8 million to $12.2 million, while the municipal hospitals' portion increased from $638,000 to over $2.2 million.

The effect of third-party reimbursement, particularly Medicaid, is further revealed by an analysis of the cost data compiled by hospitals. The difficulty of defining the hospital's product, coupled with the accounting problems in allocating its large overhead, has led hospitals to distribute costs in a manner which would facilitate their being reimbursed, that is, to inpatient care.

From 1962 through 1965 the average cost per emergency room visit for municipal hospitals fluctuated around $8.00. However, coincident with the Medicaid program it jumped to over $10.50 in 1967. This increase was probably at least in part a response to the availability of third-party reimbursement. Such an increase reinforces the belief that in the past outpatient department and emergency room costs were shifted to the maximum extent possible onto inpatient costs, since these were more generally subject to third-party reimbursement.

As third-party reimbursement is broadened to include inpatient, outpatient, and emergency room medical care, decisions about allocating resources and accounting for costs between ambulatory and inpatient care will be on firmer ground.

In short, the effect of Medicaid was twofold: first, it shifted a significant portion of emergency room users and their accompanying money flows to the offices of private physicians; second, it shifted a large proportion of patients from the emergency rooms of municipal hospitals to those of voluntary hospitals.

THE EMERGENCY ROOM:

ORGANIZATIONAL STEPCHILD IN THE

HOSPITAL STRUCTURE

Social and economic forces—the growing dependence of many people, especially the poor, on hospitals for routine medical care and the expanded financial aid controlled by policies made outside of hospitals—have led most hospitals to react passively, rather than planfully. There appears to be no city-wide planning with respect to defining the function of the emergency room or helping emergency rooms to cope with their increased patient loads, nor has there apparently been much planning by the individual hospital. Financing, staffing, and management of emergency rooms appear to be less the result of planned decisions than *ad hoc* adaptations.

Three related factors account for the hospitals' apparently passive reaction: the emergency room's nebulous position in the hospital's structure; the ambivalence of trustees, medical staffs, and administrators about quality emergency room care; the outpatient department–emergency room relationship. An even more general consideration may be the absence of effective consumer leverage.

The emergency room is an organizational stepchild. It is not a department and it does not have the weight of a department in fighting for support and resources. Unlike other departments, the emergency room is horizontally organized, that is, it tends to borrow staff and equipment from other departments.

Consequently the emergency room does not typically have much staff of its own. However, the data on staffing of emergency rooms are suspect. The statistics have grossly underestimated the number of personnel working in emergency rooms. The United Hospital Fund's reports for the voluntary hospitals,[8] which are the best available, appear to have underestimated emergency room personnel primarily because, as noted above, hospitals tend to allocate most of their emergency room costs to inpatient services to facilitate reimbursement.

Even under this policy, voluntary hospitals reported a doubling of full-time equivalent staff in emergency rooms, from 289 to 602 between 1961 and 1966. This 108 percent increase in personnel is high when considered in conjunction with the 33 percent increase in emergency room visits. However, the disaggregated statistics tell a different story: records of eight out of 45 voluntary hospitals show no personnel in their emergency rooms in 1961, while in fact these eight hospitals accounted for over 18 percent of all visits to emergency rooms during that year.

We have no way of knowing the true situation. One reasonable hypothesis is that many emergency room services were originally under the administration of the outpatient department.

With increased availability of third-party payments for emergency room care, improvements in reporting true staffing costs have occurred. The 1967 data show that only two hospitals still reported no personnel in their emergency rooms. Also the average number of full-time equivalent personnel per hospital rose from 6.2 in 1961 to 13.2 in 1967. To what extent these figures represent a change in staffing or a change in reporting cannot be ascertained.

Changes in the emergency room staffing patterns for paramedicals as well as for physicians have been piecemeal, responsive to the increased demands placed upon the services of personnel. No planning has been undertaken to forecast and/or meet future needs. As the waiting room congestion mounts and as the staff becomes harassed, the hospital administration is forced to add additional personnel, that is, physicians, nurse's aides, etc.

The possibility should be entertained that this system of *ad hoc* staffing adjustments may have a feedback effect, thereby increasing demand for emergency room services even further. When a hospital hires more staff because the increased volume of visits has reached a point where patients and staff balk, the resulting improvement in conditions may stimulate even further use of emergency room facilities. Despite earlier evidence of consumer dissatisfaction and powerlessness in the absence of suitable alternatives, the demand for emergency room services may nevertheless increase.

Interviews have indicated that throughout the city the use of salaried physicians in emergency rooms, both full and part time, has increased substantially over the past few years. This increase seems due primarily to the unwillingness of regular hospital staff to cover the emergency room, coupled with a shortage of interns and residents in the New York City hospitals, particularly in municipal hospitals. Staffing shortages were aggravated in 1962 by the New York State Code, which, by tightening the physician licensing requirements, removed most of the unlicensed foreign-trained physicians from the city's emergency rooms. Until then, foreign-trained physicians had been staffing many of the city's emergency rooms while studying for their licensing exams.

In the teaching hospitals, a staffing pattern which is gaining widespread acceptance is one in which a full-time physician supervises interns and residents, usually during the day shift, with full-time physicians employed to cover the night and/or weekend shifts and with part-time physicians working at other times during the week.

In many municipal hospitals, the physician staffing of the emergency room is tied to the affiliation system. Interviews with officials of both municipal and voluntary hospitals joined in an affiliation arrangement reveal that the emergency room has received priority. However, the affiliating voluntary hospital has considered the emergency room primarily as a chance to rotate interns and residents in its various teaching programs through a meaningful and rewarding experience—more diverse and in certain respects more challenging than conventional hospital care. And this practice has not necessarily led to improved patient care in the emergency room.

Since the emergency room's chief resource—its staff—has until recently been drawn entirely from the other medical departments within the hospital, the emergency room director, if the hospital had one, had little independence. He was forced to depend on others. While the staffing picture is changing slowly, most directors still lack the authority required to obtain the resources they need for the efficient operation of the emergency room.

One innovation which is gaining wide acceptance is the appointment of an emergency room subcommittee of the Medical Board. This practice allows the emergency room director a voice in the hospital's decision-making body, thus strengthening his ability to command resources, and has opened an important channel through which he can operate.

Recent recognition of the need for emergency room committees was seen in Commissioner Joseph Terenzio's memorandum of April, 1968, which instructed all municipal hospitals to appoint such standing committees and which mandated that all hospitals with more than 50,000 emergency room visits per year (which includes all but two) appoint a full-time director for emergency room services.

On the administrative side, the relations of the emergency room to the major departments which control personnel, equipment, and funds must be clarified, as must the responsibilities of those departments for enabling the emergency room to carry out its priority functions. But this concept has yet to be fully accepted by many governing boards, hospital administrators, and medical staffs.

MEDICAL BOARD AMBIVALENCE ABOUT
QUALITY EMERGENCY ROOM CARE

To date, hospital trustees, medical staffs, and administrators have different concepts of the role of the emergency room. Many feel that the emergency room should limit its services to emergencies, while others see the emergency room as a walk-in clinic for all types of patients. The latter group envisions the emergency room as an integral part of the hospital that should provide broad medical care for the community. A third view would be to explore alternative ambulatory care facilities which would provide more responsive services.

Those who believe that an emergency room should care only for true emergencies feel that a program of public education is required to inhibit faulty utilization and abuse. They argue that the continuing adaptations of the emergency rooms to the increased demands of nonemergency patients will result in their gradual conversion into large impersonal health supermarkets—ill adapted to provide either emergency services or general ambulatory care.

Differences in conception pervade the medical boards of many hospitals. The tendency of certain medical boards to restrict the use of the emergency room may reflect the fact that they are dominated by private practitioners who do not wish to see the emergency room develop into a substitute for the physician's office. Thus, while these boards desire to maintain a level of adequate care in the emergency room, they do not want the care to become "too good" and thereby provide direct competition to the neighborhood physician.

Such views, as well as those which favor the broad expansion and improvement of emergency room services, are an extension of the differences among medical and lay leaders that have evolved in recent years over the proper role for the hospital, and more particularly its responsibility for providing ambulatory care services for low-income persons who have limited access to private physicians.

The important point is not disagreement about the abstract role of an emergency room but rather how far municipal and voluntary hospitals should develop emergency room services. While it is difficult to prove, there is an impression that municipal hospitals have accepted the growing role of the emergency room, while voluntary hospitals remain strongly divided on the issue, a division reflected in part by the tighter triage (screening) systems for patients in voluntary hospitals.

Moreover, voluntary hospitals appear to be much more zealous in their billing and collection procedures. Until the start of Medicaid, no billings were made for emergency room visits in municipal hospitals. Even now, all that the law requires is that billings be made; it does not stipulate that the city must collect on such bills to be eligible for reimbursement from Medicaid and Medicare patients. At present, billing is done by each hospital separately. However, the procedure of billing patients not covered by Medicaid has been a failure, since few responded. In fact, some 30 percent of the bills are returned stamped "wrong address" across the front. For the municipal hospitals the time spent on billing and follow-up seems questionable if not wasteful.

Although detailed data are lacking, interviews have revealed that voluntary hospitals are much more successful in obtaining reimbursement from patients. In fact, some hospitals have employed outside collection agencies.

The philosophy still prevails that it is the hospital's obligation to provide medical care without regard to the patient's ability to pay. Nevertheless, all hospital administrations, municipal as well as voluntary, act on the belief that if there is third-party reimbursement, they should get "a piece of the action." Even with increased revenues, the emergency room will remain a money-losing operation until users or third parties are able and willing to pay full costs. At present, administrators can merely try to minimize the loss.

EMERGENCY ROOM—OUTPATIENT DEPARTMENT RELATIONSHIP

In most New York City hospitals the outpatient department and the emergency room are operated as two separate units. They have separate administrative and professional staffs, separate records systems, and separate facilities. It has been said by many that the emergency room and the outpatient department are, in fact, two separate clinics, run at different times of the day, with different staffs, and with different philosophies of medical care.

In recent years serious thought has been given to combining the outpatient department and the emergency room into a single unit. There are strong arguments both for and against this proposal.

Since most hospitals in New York City utilize two sets of administrative and professional staffs to operate their emergency rooms and outpatient departments, and since both have different admission policies, different records systems, and different philosophies of medical care, they are more frequently at odds than in agreement. Nevertheless, the same patients frequently utilize both the emergency room and the outpatient department. Thus a single unit might make it easier to provide more comprehensive round-the-clock coverage for the same population group.

However, such comprehensive care may be more than is needed. As one study has shown, many who use the emergency room do not require extensive services.[9] At the most they need the services of a physician for a minor, acute problem. The administrative choice need not be limited to the continuing independence or merger of the emergency room and the outpatient department. An important third option which the City of New York is beginning to exercise is the free-standing community clinic geared to provide first-level ambulatory services to all persons in a low-income area. This effort is directed toward overcoming many of the inadequacies in organization and service identified earlier which grow out of the limited responsiveness of the hospital to meeting ambulatory care needs.

To sum up, ambulatory patients in New York City's hospitals seem to utilize medical care in two different ways. One group needs care for chronic long-term illness and turns occasionally to the emergency room for an unexpected short-term problem. This group uses primarily the outpatient department. The other group requires episodic medical care for short-term illnesses, accidents, etc.; the emergency room is their primary source of care.

The creation of a single ambulatory unit would probably help to solve many of the organizational and administrative problems in both the emergency room and the outpatient department, but it would not automatically provide better medical care. Ambulatory patients still need care for both acute and chronic conditions and the success of a single unit would depend upon its ability to provide both.

SUMMARY

The key findings of this chapter follow:

1. New York City's emergency rooms in both voluntary and municipal hospitals passively adapted their resources to the increased demand for emergency room care. They have done little planning to fit the emergency room into the broad spectrum of services that the hospital provides.

2. The *ad hoc* hospital response to exploitation of immediately available ambulatory care by the public is an example of consumer influence through utilization upon decision-making affecting the allocation of resources.

3. The shift of patients from municipal hospitals to voluntary hospitals after Medicaid apparently indicates their preference for treatment at the latter. Furthermore, Medicaid led to a shift in the locus of services sought by the poor from emergency rooms to the offices of private physicians.

4. Reimbursement patterns and levels have played a significant role in increasing the demand for emergency room services and in the allocation of the demand among competing providers.

5. Increased staff has not stimulated the demand for emergency room services. Rather, staffing changes have been responsive to increased demands.

6. The attitudes of management (governing boards and administrators) and the framework within which the emergency room departments operate have been obstacles to improved emergency room services.

7

AMBULATORY
SERVICES

A TRADITIONAL sct of beliefs has guided the provision of care for
ambulatory patients in the United States. According to this assumption, most families obtain their needed medical care from a local
physician. Individuals are free to choose their primary doctor and
professionals are free to locate where they please. The intended
result is that each family has a physician in the community who
meets its recurrent needs.

The role of government is limited according to this philosophy:
mental health aside, public agencies serve three purposes—sanitation
and environmental control, prevention of the spread of communicable diseases, and provision of care for the poor. Local health
departments usually execute the preventive function. They test
water supplies, carry out immunization programs, examine school
children, and engage in numerous other activities designed to secure
the physical well-being of all citizens. Medical care for the poor has
been viewed as a dimension of public assistance. In times of the
"poorhouse," the sick poor were isolated and cared for there. In New
York City, special hospitals were built to care for the indigent. As
the nation moved to a system of "outdoor relief" (cash allowances
for the indigent rather than institutional confinement) under the
Social Security Act of 1935, little attention was paid to the provision
of medical care. It was not until 1950 that Congress passed a
program of federal support of vendor medical payments which had
been explicitly denied reimbursement before then. Consequently,
there developed a limited system of conventional medical care for
the poor who until then had had access only to institutional services:

the outpatient departments of teaching hospitals maintained to provide medical students and interns experience with diverse conditions which they were likely to encounter in practice, and a variety of free-standing dispensaries organized early in the century and concentrated in the low-income sections of the community. Ambulatory services received little professional attention and were almost a residual function of municipal and voluntary hospitals. Charity and the limited resources of local government paid for the care of the ambulatory sick.

The expansion of scientific knowledge and accompanying changes in the practice of medicine have made the traditional pattern of providing ambulatory care unsatisfactory for both indigent and nonindigent patients. It is now common practice for physicians to specialize and as a result families can no longer rely upon a single physician to attend to all of their medical needs. In 1966 less than 4,000 of the more than 22,000 physicians in New York City were in private general practice. It is not unlikely that an average family with children will utilize an internist, obstetrician, pediatrician, ophthalmologist, and allergist to meet its recurrent medical needs.

Care for the indigent is likely to be even more fragmented. Hospital clinics are organized according to medical specialties and subspecialties, so that a patient may have to visit several clinics to receive attention for different complaints or conditions. Moreover, the traditional distinction between preventive and therapeutic services dictates that the local health department provide a smallpox vaccination and a physical examination in school, but if a child has an acute condition the department's physician will refer him to another facility.

To overcome increasing fragmentation in the provision of care for all income groups, the traditional philosophy of ambulatory care has been reformulated. The goal of comprehensive care has been added. For those who had previously relied upon private physicians one answer is to join a group plan for medical care, preferably on a prepaid basis. Proposals for the reform of public facilities have suggested structures which will coordinate preventive, diagnostic, and curative services. With few exceptions, planned changes in the provision of ambulatory care during the 1960s were efforts to implement this goal of comprehensive care.

TRADITIONAL SOURCES OF
AMBULATORY CARE

Before presenting a discussion of reform efforts we will consider the status of the traditional sources of ambulatory care in New York City during the last decade. The figures in Table 7.1 indicate the trends in modern medical practice. When the supply of physicians

TABLE 7.1

Physicians in New York City, 1959 and 1966

	1959		1966	
	Number	Percent	Number	Percent
Physicians not in private practice				
Interns and residents	2,927	15.8	5,557	25.0
Others	1,610	8.8	3,596	16.2
Total	4,537	24.6	9,153	41.2
Physicians in private practice				
Specialists	7,807	42.2	9,269	41.6
General practitioners	6,128	33.2	3,819	17.2
Total	13,935	75.4	13,088	58.8
All physicians	18,472	100.0	22,241	100.0

Source: Nora Piore and Sandra Sokol, *A Profile of Physicians in the City of New York before Medicare and Medicaid* (Urban Research Center, Hunter College, New York, 1968).

in 1959 is compared with that in 1966 two changes become obvious. First, there are fewer doctors in private practice and the number not in private practice has doubled. Second, of those in private practice more than two-thirds were specialists in 1966. When we add to these data the fact that almost one-third of the general practitioners are over sixty-five, and that well over 80 percent of graduating medical students plan to specialize, it becomes evident that the local "family physician" will soon be a rarity. For higher-income groups this trend is counteracted to a limited extent by formally certified internists who are assuming the role of family physician, avoiding categorically only pediatrics and obstetrics.

With regard to organized ambulatory care, we find that there are several kinds of structures providing services. The clinics of over eighty voluntary and municipal hospitals are the primary source of care in New York City. About nine million visits are made to the emergency rooms and outpatient departments (OPD) of these hospitals each year. Because the emergency room is the subject of a separate chapter it will not be considered here. The number and distribution of OPD visits in 1958 and 1967 are presented in Table 7.2.

TABLE 7.2

Hospital Outpatient Department Visits in New York City

| | 1958 | | 1967 | | 1958 to 1967 |
	Number	*Percent*	*Number*	*Percent*	*Percent of Change*
Municipal hospitals	2,646,615	48.6	3,428,153	54.6	+29.5
Voluntary hospitals	2,799,094	51.4	2,853,140	45.4	+ 1.9
Total	5,445,709	100.0	6,281,293	100.0	+15.3

Sources: The 1958 figures are from Herbert Klarman, *Hospital Care in New York City* (New York: Columbia University Press, 1963) p. 34; the 1967 figures are from Health and Hospital Planning Council of Southern New York, "Ambulatory Visits by Hospital" (mimeographed, March, 1968), p. 1. The above figures for 1967 differ from those in Table 6.1 of chapter 6, because a different source was used. However, the small differences do not alter the conclusions in either chapter.

The most important fact which emerges from these data is that almost all growth in OPD services since 1958 has taken place in the municipal hospitals, continuing an antecedent trend. The absence of significant expansion in the OPD services of voluntary hospitals is explained by three factors. First, the academically oriented physicians and chiefs of service who were becoming an increasing proportion of the voluntary hospital staffs viewed the OPD as relatively uninteresting and unimportant. They preferred to devote their time and attention to the care of inpatients. Specialists, residents, and interns regarded the OPD as an undesirable assignment. Second, the OPD population differed significantly from the inpatient population. Voluntary hospital physicians care for their private patients during their stay as inpatients, while there are few private patients in the OPD.

Equally important was the fact that outpatient services were not adequately financed. Prior to the passage of Medicaid the New York City Department of Welfare paid a maximum of $7.00 per visit for patients receiving public assistance. This was generally insufficient to cover the costs of the visit. Even patients whose income was above the cut-off point for assistance could not afford to pay a charge sufficient to cover full costs. Blue Cross has permitted voluntary hospitals to include the net costs of their OPD in the calculation for per diem reimbursement for inpatient care. However, non-teaching hospitals could include only a limited amount. In addition, voluntary hospitals were reimbursed by Blue Cross for fewer than 60 percent of their inpatients so that they generally failed to recover the full cost of the OPD. The result was that the OPD service was a deficit operation for the hospital. One expert estimated that in 1965 voluntary hospitals in the metropolitan area suffered a deficit of almost $23 million in their clinic services. Because the voluntary hospital's OPD lost money, did not serve private patients, and was of little interest to the staff, it remained stagnant.

The growth of municipal OPD services is explained by circumstances similar to those described in the study of the emergency room in chapter 6. The changing demographic patterns, the declining number of physicians in poorer neighborhoods, and inadequate financing for alternative services, which account for the unplanned growth of emergency rooms, also explain the increasing load on the OPDs of the city's hospitals. As with the emergency room, consumer dissatisfaction with the quality and the conditions of municipal outpatient services has grown, and was clearly manifest in a distinct shift to private physicians and voluntary hospital clinics when these options became available through Medicaid and Medicare.

The numerous clinics operated by the New York City Department of Health are another important source of ambulatory care. Data on the attendance at various Health Department programs and clinics are presented in Table 7.3. In accordance with the traditional philosophy, the Department's activities have focused on preventive and diagnostic treatment and many programs are designed especially for children. Almost half the services provided directly by the Department fall within its school health program. Children are given polio vaccine and tested for tuberculosis. A physical examina-

TABLE 7.3

Health Department Services

	1961	1967
Clinics		
Child health	480,646	519,274
Dental	434,071	480,513
Eye	70,008	61,580
Working paper	108,729	116,606
Social hygiene	133,599	158,512
Tuberculosis	246,503	289,081
Cardiac	4,132	3,866
Nutrition	38,173	21,108
Cancer	11,604	11,630
Tropical diseases	31,693	34,558
Anti-rabies	32,990	76,494
Orthopedic	426	1,455
Other clinics	39,793	40,182
Total	1,632,367	1,814,859
School services		
Examinations	250,578	345,215
Tests and immunization	447,114	476,545
Other attention	1,048,346	981,988
Total	1,746,038	1,803,748
Total (clinic and school)	3,378,405	3,618,607

Source: Data supplied by Bureau of Records and Statistics, Department of Health, City of New York.

tion either by a private physician or by a school doctor is mandatory for all children when they enter school and once again during their school years. The Health Department gives special examinations at schools and at clinics for teenagers requiring working papers. Youngsters are given dental care at the dental clinics operated in each of the city's health districts. Preschool children are cared for at the nearly 100 child health stations or "well-baby clinics" operated by the Department. As Table 7.3 indicates, the school, child health, dental, and other services designed for children account for over two-thirds of the Department's direct provision of health services.

In general, Health Department facilities utilized by adults are either diagnostic or are aimed at the control of communicable diseases. There are clinics for the detection and treatment of tuberculosis, diagnostic services for tropical diseases, and cancer detection clinics. In addition to the direct provision of services to children and adults the Department is also responsible for enforcing the local health codes and maintaining records and vital statistics.

The data on Health Department services for 1961 and 1967 reveal no dramatic or unexpected changes. There has been a slow growth in the volume of most services. In 1967 some important innovations were begun in an effort to move toward an expanded goal of combined therapeutic and preventive care, and they will be discussed in a later section.

The free-standing clinics operated by voluntary organizations in New York City, survivors of the earlier dispensary movement, are the third traditional source of organized ambulatory care. There is no convenient, comprehensive, and accurate source of statistics for these facilities. A directory published by the Community Council of Greater New York lists about twenty organizations maintaining free-standing clinics which provide physical, as distinct from mental, health services. A sizable majority provide only dental and/or eye care. Actually independent clinics provide a substantial portion of dental care, which is only minimally represented at hospital OPDs. Clinics which do not provide eye or dental services usually provide diagnosis or treatment of a specific disease or are designed to provide general medical examinations. In comparison with the more than six million OPD visits and three million Health Department services, this score of independent clinics accounts for only a small segment of the total supply of ambulatory care services.

Two other forms of organized care for ambulatory patients, designed for closed employee populations, should be mentioned: union health centers and occupational (or industrial) medical services, the one consumer-oriented, the other responding essentially to industry need with some spill-over benefits for the individual.

Not unexpectedly, union plans have moved toward an objective of more comprehensive service for their membership in contradistinction to industrial medicine, which has a clearly restricted mission, intended to supplement rather than provide ongoing personal health care for its constituency. Although there are no definitive figures for services currently provided by the industrial sector, we can safely estimate well over a million eligibles for these two noninstitutional medical functions, with modest overlap of populations.

Originating with the provision of physical examinations dictated by safety requirements in specific industries with a considerable public risk, and with the need for occasional emergency care, in-plant medical facilities have been extended from production industries to white-collar services and business firms. Prior to the 1960s, industrial medical departments in New York were limited to the modest number of large employers within the city—principally utilities, insurance, the Federal Reserve Bank, department stores—but with the development in the last decade of midtown office space housing large employee concentrations, there has been a proliferation of these facilities. In the absence of any hard data, we estimate the current number of units at about 200 in and around New York City and the number is expected to increase concomitantly with the further expansion of national corporate headquarters in the central business district.

Organization and range of services are fairly uniform. The modal facility is staffed by a medical director, several full-time physicians, a number of part-time consultants, and nurses, supported by laboratory and X-ray technicians and clerical personnel. It has a tripartite program consisting of mandatory preemployment examinations, voluntary periodic examinations and consultative services for employees, and emergency treatment as required by employees and office visitors. To supplement the last service, there may be an arrangement with a nearby voluntary hospital. Occasionally dentistry is included. To avoid any suspicion of competition with private practice, ongoing treatment is fastidiously avoided, services are not available to dependents, and facilities operate only during working hours. If additional procedures are indicated, individuals are referred to their community physician; follow-up is more or less conscientiously pursued. Some firms require an employee to report to the medical department following a specified period of absence from work. Currently, the chief contribution of this fairly extensive group of facilities is their diagnostic and consultation services, the value of which is ultimately determined by the availability (physically and financially) and the quality of subsequent service. Slippage that occurs between screening and adequate treatment is an inherent deficiency of independent limited-function facilities.

The vast majority of firms in New York City are not of a size to justify elaborate facilities of the type described. Smaller businesses which have a screening and examination program may refer executives and employees to similar privately owned clinics, of which there are approximately twenty at the present time. Beekman Hospital, in a move to dovetail its services with the changing needs of the surrounding community, is in the process of setting up a unit to accommodate downtown firms. Less elaborate private groups, generally offering physician services only, are located in central buildings in the various occupational districts of the city to perform examinations and emergency care; as private practice groups, they do not avoid continuing treatment. At least one independent unit is planned for the World Trade Center now under construction.

More modest plants contract in a variety of ways for the provision chiefly of emergency services. A recent interesting approach has been the introduction of a joint program sponsored by Brookdale Hospital and the Visiting Nurse Service for regular visits to small plants in Brooklyn; services here are directed at employees who are otherwise poorly connected to any health resource.

To gain some precise data on the existence, magnitude, and scope of occupational health services, the Division of Industrial Hygiene of the State Department of Labor is currently undertaking a survey via mailed questionnaires of all plants employing 100 individuals or more. A similar inquiry in 1967 failed to yield a statistically adequate response; with a considerably simplified schedule, the desired data may be obtained.

More comprehensive medical care, rather than limited in-plant health services, is provided to employees in some of the city's highly organized industries. While generally referred to as "union health centers," these programs include facilities managed jointly by representatives of management and labor as well as those sponsored exclusively by trade unions. Sizable operations in New York City include the Sidney Hillman Health Center serving the Amalgamated Clothing Workers of America; the ILGWU Union Health Center; individual health centers for members of Local 32B of the Building Service Employees Union, and of Local 1205 of the Teamsters Union; and multiple facility programs operated by the Consolidated Edison Company and its Employees' Mutual Aid Society, and by the Union Family Medical Fund of the Hotel Industry of New York.

At these centers a broad range of diagnostic and therapeutic services is provided by well-qualified physicians, most of whom are employed on a part-time basis. More than one center provides dental care, but dental services and psychiatric care are usually excluded. Benefits were originally available only to workers and this is still the case in some programs. Others care for the employee's family as a courtesy and charge a nominal fee, and some have extended full coverage to the worker's dependents. Hospitalization arrangements vary considerably. Three facilities of the Union Family Medical Fund are located at teaching hospitals with which they have contracts providing for professional staffing and for inpatient care; the Consolidated Edison program provides a choice of thirty-six teaching and community hospitals with which it has made inpatient arrangements; the Sidney Hillman Health Center relies for hospitalization upon the individual affiliations of its medical staff. To cover hospitalization costs some unions contract with Blue Cross while others maintain their own insurance fund. Most facilities are free-standing clinics which house their own auxiliary services, but Consolidated Edison operates four clinics on company premises and three of the Union Family Medical Fund offices are located at hospitals.

Approximately three-quarters of a million people, not all of whom live within New York City, are potentially eligible for some form of care at union- or union-management-sponsored health centers. The future growth and viability of these programs will be determined by a complicated set of factors not all of which are directly related to the ability of these centers to provide adequate care. Union membership is affected by the changing economic structure of the city, which is shifting away from the traditionally well-organized industries. Changing residential patterns place many New York City workers in scattered and outlying neighborhoods. To utilize a centrally located health center an employee's family may have to make a relatively long trip. At the same time rising medical costs force families to think twice before ignoring employment-related benefits when they need medical care.

The traditional sources of ambulatory care may be categorized by the populations they serve. Private practitioners provide most of the care for those who can afford to pay a fee for service. In addition, several large unions have organized comprehensive medical centers for their members and families, and an increasing number of business and industrial firms provide more restricted diagnostic services to employees. For the indigent, preventive and screening services are provided by the Department of Health, while care for acute conditions is available at hospital OPDs. Both paying and non-paying patients face the problem of fragmented care.

REFORM EFFORTS FOR THE

MIDDLE CLASS

As we have noted, in recent years the dominant concern of reformers in the field of health services has been to overcome fragmentation and establish the provision of high-quality comprehensive care. Efforts to extend group practice, which predate the 1960s, are still the most promising way for the average citizen to overcome the difficulties arising from the increased specialization of the medical profession.

The most significant attempt to provide New Yorkers with medical care through a prepaid group practice plan is the Health Insurance Plan of Greater New York (HIP), incorporated in 1944 and operational since 1946–47. The thirty-one groups currently affiliated with this plan provide care for nearly three-quarters of a million people in the metropolitan area. While this is certainly a sizable population, the plan's growth in recent years has been limited. Figure 7.1 shows the number of persons enrolled from 1947 to 1968. It should be noted that the data for 1962 to 1966 include several thousand Old Age Assistance recipients enrolled in a demonstration program run by the New York City Welfare Department. With the advent of Medicaid this project was terminated, but the enrollees and all other Medicaid eligibles have had an opportunity to join HIP. The figures for 1966 to 1968 show no significant growth in the non-Medicaid enrollment, but reveal that over 80,000 Medicaid eligibles have chosen to receive their care from HIP groups. While HIP apparently no longer attracts many new self-supporting workers, the plan is demonstrating an ability to provide satisfactory care to a sizable number of medically indigent people.

The more than twenty years' experience of HIP provides evidence of the difficulties in establishing a prepaid group practice plan in an urban area. The most desirable form of prepaid group practice is considered to be one which is hospital-based and employs physicians on a full-time basis. HIP has not been able to meet these criteria.

The HIP groups have relied heavily on part-time physicians. As a consequence a member of a group may have to compete with the doctor's private patients. Also, while precise data are not available, both patients and administrators believe there is a higher than desirable rate of turnover among the groups' physicians. This can defeat the groups' efforts to provide members with a family physician with whom they can develop a long-term relationship.

These staffing problems have deep-rooted causes. Organized medicine has traditionally opposed any payment system other than a fee for service. Although the medical establishment in New York is more liberal than comparable bodies in other areas of the country, HIP did not begin without difficulty. When the HIP Medical Control Board was first organized in 1946, four out of the five County Medical Societies in New York City refused to send representatives. Some hospitals denied staff privileges to certain HIP doctors. Much of this hostility no longer exists, but a no less potent pressure still at work is the lure of potentially high professional incomes obtainable in an active fee-for-service practice.

Most of the HIP groups have operated without their own hospital and without even a group hospital affiliation. For inpatient services

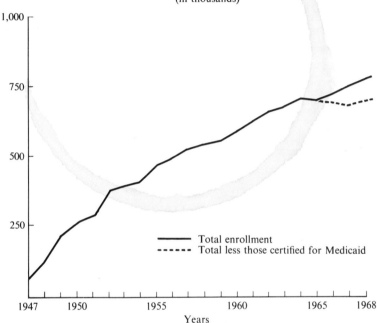

Figure 7.1. Number of Persons Enrolled in HIP, 1947-1968 (in thousands)

they have had to rely upon the staff appointment(s) of each participating physician. This dependence gives the group no central control over the bed supply available to it. The enrollee has no assurance of the quality or location of the hospital he may one day have to utilize.

Another factor which has inhibited HIP expansion is the pervasive bias in many consumers' minds against prepayment plans. People are reluctant to join a group practice plan because freedom of physician choice is considered a privilege which accompanies middle-class status. Medical care provided in an organized or group setting is regarded as suitable only for those who cannot afford an alternative.

Until recently the Montefiore Medical Group had been an HIP unit which avoided many of these difficulties. It was located in a middle-class area at a well-regarded teaching institution and employed only physicians associated full time with the hospital. However, this group encountered other difficulties and in January, 1970, terminated its contract with HIP. Because of the volume and quality of services it provided its members and because of the necessity to absorb its share of the high cost of selected hospital operations, this group had higher operating expenses than other HIP units. The hospital could no longer meet the deficit resulting from the difference between HIP capitation payments and the group's allocated costs. This fact points up another problem for HIP. It must compete with the premium rates of other insurance plans while offering comprehensive benefits. Therefore, HIP cannot make open-ended financial commitments to cover all the costs of nonprofit groups offering high-quality medical care.

One further point should be made about the HIP experience. In 1966, over 60 percent of HIP members were city employees and their families; this figure reflects a decline from earlier years. To a considerable degree HIP was originally an experiment in the delivery of medical care financed by the City of New York for its employees. The city now spends about $50 million annually for various forms of employee health insurance; this appropriation should be kept in mind along with the budget of the Health Services Administration when innovations in medical care are contemplated.

Currently, the city has under way a modest experiment to extend physician services by means of group practice to a lower middle-class area that has suffered physician attrition. As of 1969, the Mayflower Medical Group, with a complement of seventeen doctors, has been operating in Bensonhurst under a contract with the city to serve that community together with Medicaid patients from neighboring Coney Island. The incentive to the group has been the willingness of the Department of Social Services to reimburse it as a unit for Medicaid services, a departure from the general requirement to pay only the individual physician in adherence to "freedom of choice." Funded with a federal grant, an office to encourage group practice units has been set up within the Health Services Administration to develop administrative procedures, criteria for service, and incentives which will stimulate further organization by competent physicians in high-priority areas. It remains to be seen whether these groups can be made sufficiently attractive to both physicians and consumers to restore quality private practice with some degree of permanency to areas from which it has disappeared.

PROGRAMS FOR THE POOR

Long after prepaid group practice was first introduced as a remedy for fragmented care for the middle class, there developed a movement to provide comprehensive and high-quality care for the poor. The first of recent steps in this direction were the innovations at the Gouverneur Ambulatory Care Center undertaken early in the 1960s under the affiliation program of the Hospitals Department. Experiences at Gouverneur provided a model for future developments throughout the city and, even more significantly, for future developments throughout the nation under the Office of Economic Opportunity.

Gouverneur Hospital was built by New York City in 1898 to serve a portion of the Lower East Side. By the early 1950s the physical plant of the heavily utilized facility was deteriorating rapidly. It was difficult to recruit physicians, and when the New York University School of Medicine terminated a brief affiliation in 1955, the Joint Commission on the Accreditation of Hospitals withdrew accreditation. In 1961 Hospitals Commissioner Ray Trussell recommended that the hospital be closed. Local community groups objected vehemently. Eventually a compromise was reached. Outpatient services would be provided at the old building by medical staff from Beth Israel Hospital and a new hospital would be built nearby.

The ambulatory care unit began operating in 1962. The program was fortunate to attract an imaginative director, Dr. Howard Brown, who sought to provide comprehensive, high-quality care in a manner that respects the dignity of the patient and in an atmosphere that is pleasant and attractive. The entire building was redecorated, a realistic appointment system was instituted, patients were assigned a family doctor, and hard wooden benches were replaced with plastic chairs. Coordinated medical care, intensified social services, and team staffing were key points of emphasis. Local residents retained an interest in the program and Gouverneur became the first neighborhood health center, although it was not yet called by that name.

Another early effort to provide comprehensive care for the poor was initiated by the Departments of Health and Welfare in cooperation with the New York Hospital–Cornell University Medical Center. For two years, 1961 to 1963, a specially organized group of physicians, social service staff, and allied health personnel provided a wide range of inpatient and outpatient services to over 1,000 families receiving public assistance. The aim was to determine whether a comprehensive hospital-based facility could be substituted for the fragmented system of care which served the indigent. While the possibility of implementing such an arrangement was established, there were significant difficulties. Despite the fact that the patient population was drawn from the nearest welfare center, New York Hospital was farther from their homes than alternative municipal facilities. Consequently, almost 40 percent of those eligible never visited the project and those in attendance frequently received some care at other facilities. Budget was an equally important difficulty. Estimates of total costs for patients served by the project were considerably higher than those for a control group who relied upon the traditional sources of care (approximately $218 per year compared to $143 per year). Since estimates for the project's patients include costs for services provided elsewhere, it must be noted that the total would be even higher if all their care were obtained at New York Hospital. The project's brief duration did not allow for any satisfactory evaluation of the effectiveness of care, but it was observed that there were no significant differences between the study group and the controls in infant and adult mortality rates, and that there was little systematic difference in patterns of perinatal care. Because of these difficulties the project was discontinued, but it effectively demonstrated the possibility of using existing hospital facilities for comprehensive care to indigent families.

In the mid-1960s two pieces of legislation were enacted which encouraged and facilitated the development of comprehensive services for the poor—Title XIX of the Social Security Act (Medicaid) and the Economic Opportunity Act of 1964. Medicaid provided federal and state support for medical care for individuals receiving public assistance and for those classified as medically indigent. The New York State program was launched in 1966, with high hopes. The poor would now be given funds to buy into the "mainstream" of American medicine. Fees would be paid to private physicians and voluntary hospitals who treated the poor. The indigent as well as the wealthy would now be able to get their care from private physicians and one standard would prevail for all.

The simple fact is that this strategy did not work. Doctors were not available in areas where the indigent were concentrated. Most competent physicians had already moved out of the ghettos and those who remained were frequently lacking in hospital appointments and specialized skills. The fees Medicaid paid were not as high as those the physicians could charge wealthier patients, so the poor were still at a disadvantage. As data presented in our review of the emergency room indicate, the result was only a small decrease in the number of clinic visits, although there was a shift from the public to the voluntary sector. The poor continued to rely heavily upon the OPD as their primary source of care.

The Office of Economic Opportunity (OEO) staff took a different approach. Soon after the War on Poverty was initiated, it became evident that medical care should be an important part of this effort. Entry into training or employment usually requires a medical examination and often the poor need remedial treatment. In addition, examinations of children enrolled in Headstart programs revealed grave deficiencies in health care. Because of these unmet needs an amendment to the Economic Opportunity Act was passed in 1966 which earmarked over $50 million for neighborhood health centers.

The neighborhood health center program soon became the focus of medical reform. The physical structure would be concrete evidence that the OEO was acting for the poor. The center would also be a source of jobs for local residents and could be used as a base for community activity. Professionals who advocated reform of the occupational and organizational structure of medicine looked upon the program as an opportunity to demonstrate important innovations. By August, 1968, there were forty-eight centers throughout the nation receiving OEO funds; by August, 1969, seven were operating in New York City.

The OEO centers have given comprehensive care a broad definition. A complete medical clinic, a dental clinic, an eye clinic, simple laboratory services, and even a pharmacy are frequently contained within the facility. In addition, other functions are being performed by the centers. Training programs are conducted for community residents to prepare them as allied medical workers. Many centers serve as a base for organizing action groups to fight for improvements in housing, sanitation, and welfare services.

While there is probably no such thing as a "typical" neighborhood health center, a review of one center's experience may illustrate the nature of the OEO program. The Martin Luther King, Jr. Neighborhood Health Center, originally known as the Montefiore Neighborhood Medical Care Demonstration, began operating with funds received from the OEO in June, 1967. In the summer of 1968 the operation moved from a storefront to a new five-story facility. The center is intended to serve a 55-square-block area of about 45,000 people in the South Bronx. About 95 percent of this population are either Negro or Puerto Rican. They are characterized by a low average family income, a high infant mortality rate, and a high incidence of tuberculosis, and they include a large number of drug addicts.

Montefiore Hospital became interested in the area as a result of its affiliation with Morrisania Hospital, the local municipal hospital.

Since 1962 Montefiore has provided staff for Morrisania under a contract with the City of New York. For reasons discussed elsewhere in this volume, the emergency room and clinics at Morrisania were being used by residents of the area as a primary source of medical care. The staff believed that a neighborhood health center providing comprehensive ambulatory services would improve the care available and relieve Morrisania's overburdened facilities.

The center's program has four components. Preventive and curative medical services are provided to families. The staff is organized into teams consisting of an internist, pediatrician, dentist, and one or more nurses and family health workers. The last-named are recruited from the neighborhood. Each family is assigned to a team which is responsible for its total care. Specialists are available for consultation and hospitalization is provided at either Montefiore or Morrisania. In addition to providing family medical care the center conducts a training program. Local residents are trained for family health worker positions in the center and for allied health positions in other facilities. There is a community development program which works with a twenty-one-member community advisory board. Lawyers on the center's staff work with community groups. They provide legal advice to local organizations and train health workers in legal skills. Finally, there is a research and evaluation unit which seeks to assess the impact of the project.

The OEO program has encountered its share of problems. In 1966 the American Medical Association (AMA), offering unsolicited advice, urged abandonment of these new efforts in medical care. The leadership felt that Medicaid provided an adequate federal program for helping the poor more acceptable to the AMA because of Medicaid's guarantee of freedom of choice to the consumer and of fee-for-service to the physician. The AMA also warned that, since the centers employ a high quotient of professional manpower, staffing an extensive network of neighborhood facilities would prove difficult. Since then, however, the AMA has become more sensitized to the growing demands of the urban poor. In 1969 its officials, publicly no less than privately, acknowledged grave deficiencies in the system and recommended to the profession that it assume greater community responsibility. They warned that significant changes in health care delivery were inevitable, with or without organized medical support. And they recommended that the nation's physicians assume an active role in innovative efforts to extend and improve medical services to the vast deprived segment of the population.

Many of the newly established centers have advanced the lure of social adventure and experimentation and have been able to elicit the support of some teaching hospitals to assist them in recruiting. As the glamour wears off, securing medical manpower may become a serious problem. The centers have also proved to be considerably more expensive than was originally anticipated. Annual costs of about $250 per person, exclusive of hospitalization, have been encountered at some centers in New York City offering a broad spectrum of services. To provide care for all the nation's poor at such a rate would require a magnitude of expenditures which the federal budget cannot reasonably be expected to absorb. Finally, OEO programs have had internal difficulties arising from conflicts among community representatives, allied health employees, hospital administration, and the medical staff. No ideal combination of roles has yet been discovered for such diverse groups.

In response to the unequivocal deficiencies of ambulatory care as provided by emergency rooms and hospital OPDs, and to community groups' demands for increased participation in health planning and operations, the city undertook an ambitious program to restructure and decentralize its health system.

Based on its own Gouverneur experience and the ambitious goals of the OEO centers, and using funds available through the New York State Medicaid program, the New York City Health Services Administration undertook in 1967 a program of neighborhood family care centers (NFCC). The director of the Gouverneur project was elevated by the mayor to the dual position of Health Services Administrator and Commissioner of Health. Under his administration plans were made for a system of about thirty centers throughout the city which would provide comprehensive care for those in need. The units would be built by renovating and adding to existing health centers, by adding to hospitals under construction, and by providing new free-standing facilities. Several large centers were to incorporate community mental health facilities under the joint administration of the New York City Community Mental Health Board and the New York City Health Department. The total capital investment was estimated to be about $100 million. As envisaged, the system would serve both the self-supporting and the indigent populations. The planning, administration, and operation of each unit were to involve the participation of neighborhood residents.

Once the centers were established it was anticipated that operating funds would be provided through Medicaid reimbursements. The NFCCs were expected to be almost completely self-supporting. However, in order for that to happen some changes in pricing were required. The Health Department facilities traditionally offered their services free of charge. To put them on a sound financial basis the state legislature enacted the Ghetto Medicine Bill in 1968. Local public health officials were authorized to charge fees for clinic services and to collect them from the local social service department through the state Medicaid program. The statute also permitted the local health departments to compromise or waive the collection of fees for those who were not eligible for Medicaid and the state would provide funds to meet half of the resultant deficit. This arrangement avoided the necessity of charging patients who used public facilities fees for services they formerly received free and which poorer individuals still received free under Medicaid. However, the potential of the Ghetto Medicine Bill as a source of funds for ambulatory care was never realized. The state legislature appropriated only minimal amounts for the program and the city found itself competing with voluntary agencies for the funds. When the legislature placed a freeze on Medicaid reimbursement rates in 1969, several voluntary hospitals found themselves short of funds and threatened to close their OPDs because of the deficits these services generated. To prevent such closures Ghetto Medicine Bill money was diverted to the voluntary hospitals and the city's program could no longer depend upon this source of funds.

New York's ambitious program to establish neighborhood family care centers throughout the city was scarcely off the drawing board when it was undermined by Medicaid cutbacks at the state and federal levels as early as 1968. These did not affect such capital planning as had occurred, which was directed toward the construction of several new facilities and the renovation and conversion of specific district health centers for general care. A physical and functional model, to be replicated throughout the system, had also been devised, adaptable to the smaller general care centers and to the larger facilities incorporating community mental health services as well. On the operational side, planning had also proceeded far enough to designate supporting hospitals that would provide specialty care and inpatient services for the neighborhood centers. A limited number of staffing contracts were being negotiated with selected teaching hospitals to provide competent professional personnel and supervision.

The critical issue of manpower planning took several new directions. A basic concept was the introduction of OEO-pioneered staffing patterns, involving the utilization of a considerably higher proportion of allied health workers relative to professional personnel. These ancillary workers were to be drawn to a large extent from the neighborhood. As far as feasible the center also looked forward to recruiting unskilled individuals for assignments requiring a limited amount of on-the-job training that would constitute a first step toward a health career. These local workers were expected to facilitate the access and attachment of neighborhood residents to the center and enhance utilization of its services.

Finally, with respect to professional staff, the most critically deficient component in the poverty areas, it was hoped that the neighborhood care program would engage the growing social concern of medical students and residents sufficiently to work in the family care centers, at least for a period of several years. It must be mentioned that planning for the program of ambulatory care under the vigorous direction of Dr. Mary McLaughlin, then Assistant Health Commissioner, encountered both internal challenges from traditionalists who opposed deviation of the Health Department from exclusively defined public health functions, and external challenges from local groups who used the program as a staging ground for the determination of community power.

In the presence of persisting financial strictures that are not likely to be loosened by the current federal administration and of complex manpower strategies that have yet to be implemented, the city has nonetheless committed itself to a priority program of seven NFCCs, four of which are under contract for expeditious construction by the State Health and Mental Hygiene Facilities Improvement Corporation; the remaining three will be undertaken by the Department of Public Works subject to its cumbersome administrative and operational procedures.

One family care center, slated for the Soundview area of the Bronx, is to be constructed by the Lavenberg Foundation in an unusual collaboration of the city and private philanthropy; negotiation toward a final agreement has not yet been concluded. There is little likelihood that the earliest of these innovative structures can become fully operational much before the mid-1970s since construction is not yet under way.

It is important, however, to distinguish between structural and programmatic aspects of the program. Two units located in existent district health centers are currently operational, in Bedford-Stuyvesant and in South Jamaica, in addition to two ambulatory care programs, Gouverneur and Bronx-Morrisania, initiated some years ago under the affiliation system and budgeted by the Hospitals Department. Further programmatic change more limited in scope than the original NFCC model may be anticipated in the near future. It is not irrelevant for the city's own ambulatory care planning that in 1969 a federal OEO program review recommended closer physical as well as functional relationships between health centers and existing hospital facilities for more effective service.

In sum, the city's sights for an effective health program for the poor are ambitious and will be followed with interest. However, given the time dimensions for implementation of the program and fiscal limitations, it must be recognized that existing emergency room and hospital OPD structures, for all their shortcomings, will continue to be the backbone of ambulatory service for an indefinite period. Accordingly, municipal reform efforts must be two-directional: to expedite effective implementation of NFCCs, and simultaneously to improve the hospital emergency room and OPD network.

CONCLUSION

Planned reform within a complex system characteristically adopts a single model in an effort to overcome the aggregate deficiencies of the component elements of the system and to eliminate the inevitable friction and slippage among them. It must be apparent, however, that where health services are concerned, no singular solution is desirable, much less feasible.

In seeking to structure a more responsive system of health services, attention must be directed not only to establishing new institutions but also to providing improved linkages among those in existence. As the maps on pp. 162-65 indicate, New York City already has an extensive network of ambulatory care facilities. It consists of approximately 80 municipal and voluntary hospital outpatient departments, 27 health centers operated by the Department of Health, almost 200 separate school health facilities, and many other municipal free-standing clinics including over 90 child health stations. While these facilities are located throughout the city, many are concentrated in poverty areas, the names of which are underlined on the maps.

Improvements in the existing system could make ambulatory services available to almost all those who require them. Detailed studies of each neighborhood could help pinpoint facilities which should be linked together as well as those whose services should be expanded. In some cases improved transportation, including buses run by the health agencies, might make basic services more easily accessible.

To increase the efficiency of the entire system, two types of linkages are required. Each ambulatory care facility should be affiliated with a central hospital to provide needed inpatient care and specialized manpower for consultation and treatment when required. It is unrealistic and undesirable for each neighborhood to have a hospital of its own. Second, closer ties should be established between the different health facilities and the people they serve. Indigenous personnel could be more generally employed to inform the population of available services, to ensure that appointments are kept, and to provide a channel of communication between the professionals and their clients.

Related to the need for greater coordination and responsiveness is the need for widespread implementation of the operational reforms demonstrated at OEO centers. The new techniques—uniform records, a flexible appointment system, family registration, and imaginative use of allied health manpower—should be adopted by hospital outpatient departments as well as by Health Department facilities.

Prepaid group practice, which was designed to improve the quality and reduce the costs of care for the self-supporting man and his family, has never received the acceptance necessary for basic restructuring of the health system. As long as physicians have available the more lucrative option of private practice, it will be difficult for groups to recruit and retain full-time staff. Until consumers abandon old assumptions about the inferiority of organized care, the growth in enrollment will be restricted.

Existing political and social conditions do not provide much hope for altering either of these circumstances. To use a currently fashionable term, the most "pragmatic" strategy is to experiment with health insurance plans. The inclusion of coverage for outpatient services in policies would relieve the consumer's financial burden and provide an incentive for hospitals to improve their ambulatory services. In addition, evaluations of the experience of existing group practices indicate that there are potential savings through reduced hospitalization rates and shorter length of stay when ambulatory services are included in insurance plans.

The voluntary hospitals' failure to respond to the growing need of the city's changing population, the withdrawal of private physician manpower from large sections of the city, and the lack of coordination between municipal health and hospital services have led to the proposal of a new system of comprehensive health centers similar to the OEO neighborhood demonstration projects. Extensive manpower requirements and supplementary health-related services of the OEO demonstrations have made them expensive operations. At present the city has adopted a priority program for NFCCs, but with persistent Medicaid strictures it will be faced with insufficient operating funds.

There are no easy solutions to these difficult problems, but some guide for future decisions may be suggested. To ensure reasonable costs, a balance must be struck between the limited program traditionally maintained by municipal health and hospital facilities and the extensive list of activities developed by some OEO neighborhood centers. Those planning for the city's NFCCs should adopt as a high-priority goal the development of a model for the efficient delivery of health services which can be widely replicated at reasonable costs. The desire of local leadership whose ideology calls for expanding community participation in policy determination to broaden the services at neighborhood facilities is understandable. However, it is questionable whether a tightening supply of health dollars should be relied upon to finance a wide range of social services. If the high costs of neighborhood ambulatory facilities are to be justified on the basis of their stimulation of community organization and development, the goals should be made explicit and evaluations of their effectiveness in achieving the desired ends undertaken. The results may then be compared with a variety of alternative programs which also pursue the same objectives. Planners who seriously support such objectives should give consideration to the investment of resources in agencies and programs which are directly concerned with generating these changes, rather than anticipate the secondary results from appropriations to municipal departments or grants awarded to voluntary hospitals.

Both the carrot and the stick can be employed to implement changes. Additional money and enforced regulations can be used to improve emergency rooms and OPDs. Available capital funds could be more liberally channeled into ambulatory functions through the establishment of priority goals at the level of the regional facilities planning authority. The inclusion of outpatient diagnostic procedures under health insurance programs would provide more funds. Medicare and Medicaid reimbursement for outpatient services on a cost basis continues to be crucial for OPD support.

Finally, the standards established for program review (however implemented by the new Health and Hospitals Corporation) and by the administrators of reimbursement programs could be used to improve the quality of emergency room and OPD services and reorganize them in a manner more convenient for the consumer, perhaps in conjunction, where feasible, with future OEO projects.

The NFCCs will similarly be subject to reimbursement review since they will be staffed by selected hospitals under contractual agreement with the Health Department, and eventually—although the time schedule has not been specified—with the Health and Hospitals Corporation.

Over-all, the most critical challenge for the city lies in the development of new and effective controls to maximize the quality and quantity of services yielded in return for its large investment in ambulatory care.

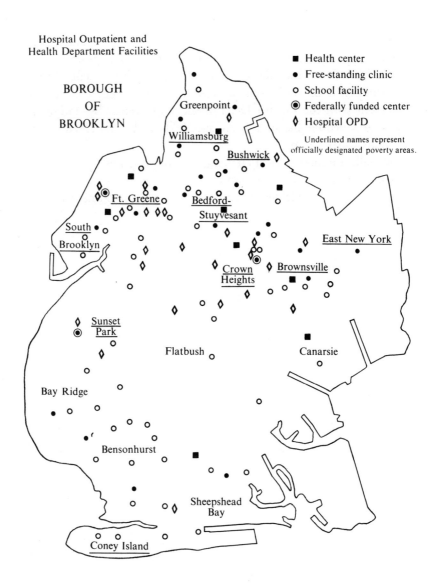

Hospital Outpatient and
Health Department Facilities

BOROUGH
OF
BROOKLYN

Greenpoint

Williamsburg

Bushwick

Ft. Greene

Bedford-
Stuyvesant

South
Brooklyn

East New York

Crown
Heights

Brownsville

Sunset
Park

Flatbush

Canarsie

Bay Ridge

Bensonhurst

Sheepshead
Bay

Coney Island

■ Health center
● Free-standing clinic
○ School facility
◉ Federally funded center
◊ Hospital OPD

Underlined names represent
officially designated poverty areas.

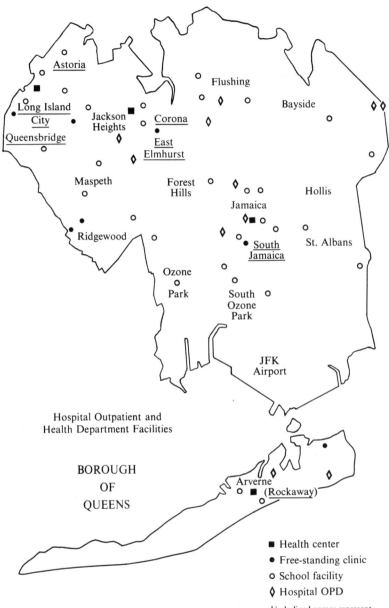

Astoria

Flushing

Long Island
City

Jackson
Heights

Corona

Bayside

Queensbridge

East
Elmhurst

Maspeth

Forest
Hills

Hollis

Jamaica

Ridgewood

South
Jamaica

St. Albans

Ozone
Park

South
Ozone
Park

JFK
Airport

Hospital Outpatient and
Health Department Facilities

BOROUGH
OF
QUEENS

Arverne
(Rockaway)

■ Health center
● Free-standing clinic
○ School facility
◊ Hospital OPD

Underlined names represent
officially designated poverty areas.

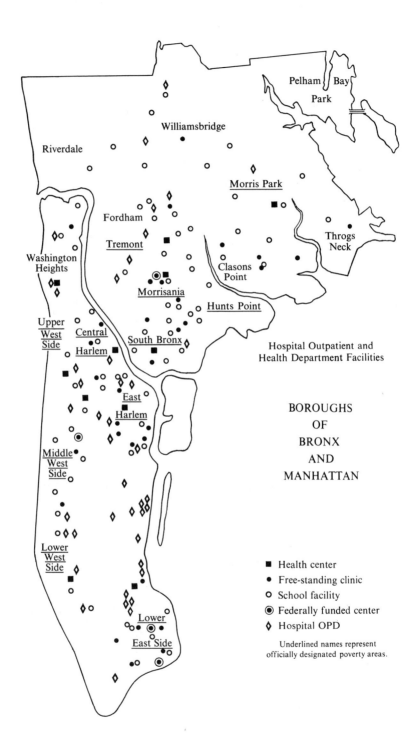

Pelham Bay Park

Williamsbridge

Riverdale

Morris Park

Throgs Neck

Fordham

Tremont

Washington Heights

Clasons Point

Morrisania

Hunts Point

Upper West Side

Central Harlem

South Bronx

Hospital Outpatient and
Health Department Facilities

East Harlem

BOROUGHS
OF
BRONX
AND
MANHATTAN

Middle West Side

Lower West Side

■ Health center
● Free-standing clinic
○ School facility
◉ Federally funded center
◊ Hospital OPD

Underlined names represent
officially designated poverty areas.

Lower East Side

Hospital Outpatient and
Health Department Facilities

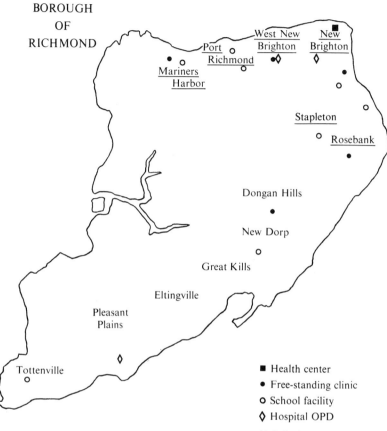

BOROUGH
OF
RICHMOND

West New
Brighton

New
Brighton

Port
Richmond

Mariners
Harbor

Stapleton

Rosebank

Dongan Hills

New Dorp

Great Kills

Eltingville

Pleasant
Plains

Tottenville

■ Health center
● Free-standing clinic
○ School facility
◊ Hospital OPD

Underlined names represent
officially designated poverty areas.

8

THE PROCESS OF REGIONALIZATION: THE BRONX

REGIONALIZATION of health services is not a new concept. Planners have long sought to rationalize the organization of medical care within a geographic area. From studies predating passage of the Hill-Burton Act to the publication of the Piel Commission Report in 1967, authorities urged that "the delivery of personal health services should be so organized as to be accessible and available to all from the point of primary service or care through the community hospital to the well-spring of medical science represented in the teaching hospital and medical school."[1] The design calls for a network of ambulatory care facilities each of which is related to a community hospital. In turn, each community hospital would be tied to the teaching hospital or medical school that serves as the regional medical center. The Piel Report represented this hierarchical or "regional" pattern diagrammatically as shown in Figure 8.1.

This definition of regionalization is undoubtedly far more comprehensive than many of the concept's supporters would deem necessary. A less systematic formulation might require only the sharing of expensive equipment and specialized units, which teaching institutions tend to accumulate, in order to avoid inefficient duplications and the assurance that everyone living in the designated region has ready access to some source of ambulatory and inpatient care. Nonetheless, the Piel Commission's comprehensive definition serves as a model which is useful in making observations and judgments about experiences in the real world.

Figure 8.1. Model of Health Services and Facilities
in a Regional Plan

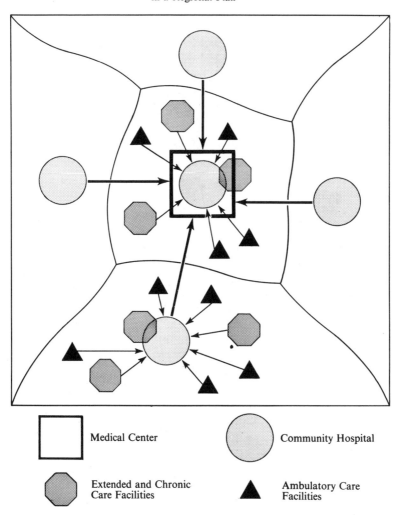

◻ Medical Center

⬤ Community Hospital

⬢ Extended and Chronic
Care Facilities

▲ Ambulatory Care
Facilities

Source: Commission on the Delivery of Personal Health Services
(Piel Commission), *Comprehensive Community Health Services for
New York City*, December, 1967, p. 27.

While there is widespread agreement that the rationalization and coordination required by such regional models is a desirable end, the planners' visions have remained difficult to implement. In this chapter we will discuss one region—the Bronx—which appears to have progressed further along these lines than others and we ask the following questions: What has made possible the degree of regionalization that exists? In what ways and for what reasons does the existing configuration deviate from the idealized model? What forces are likely to transform present patterns? In examining the process of regionalization we will seek to evaluate the role of planned intervention as distinct from other underlying factors such as demographic trends, financial pressures, and efforts at institutional enhancement in effectuating change.

Among the hospitals in the South Bronx, an area populated primarily by low-income Negroes and Puerto Ricans, is Lincoln Hospital, a 350-bed municipal facility. To the north, but still in a largely ghetto area, is the Fulton Division of the Bronx-Lebanon Hospital. Together with the Concourse Division, it constitutes the 564-bed Bronx-Lebanon Hospital Center. In the same area lies Morrisania, a 331-bed municipal facility. In the north central area adjacent to Bronx Park is Fordham, a municipal hospital with over 400 beds. To the east, just off the Hutchinson River Parkway, in proximity to each other, are the Albert Einstein College of Medicine of Yeshiva University with its 366-bed hospital, the Bronx Municipal Center with 1,208 beds, and the Bronx State Hospital for mental patients with over 1,000 beds. In the northernmost sections of the Bronx are Montefiore Hospital, the largest voluntary hospital in the borough with more than 750 beds, and Misericordia Hospital, a 330-bed voluntary institution. These are the major hospitals in the borough. They are supplemented by three other voluntary general hospitals, three voluntary long-term hospitals, and seven proprietary hospitals. There is also a Veterans Administration Hospital in the Bronx (see Figure 8.2).

These twenty-three institutions constitute all the hospitals in the Bronx, but they are surely not a single system. Rather, we should speak of the several parallel systems which exist within the Bronx. The Albert Einstein College of Medicine is responsible for provid-

Figure 8.2. Location and Relationships of Bronx Hospitals

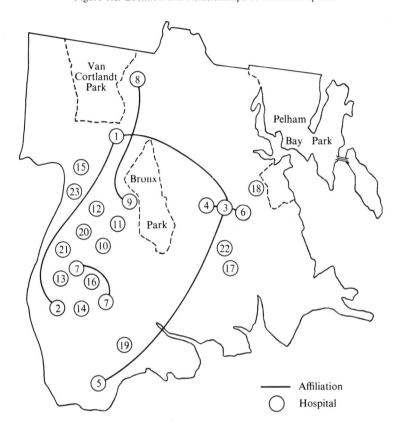

For names corresponding to numbers see Table 8.1.

ing medical personnel at three institutions. In addition to its own hospital the college faculty supervises care at the Bronx Municipal Center and at Lincoln Hospital. Montefiore is connected with Morrisania through a comprehensive affiliation contract. Montefiore is also affiliated with the Einstein College of Medicine, and in 1969 the college hospital was placed under the administrative control of Montefiore. Hence we can speak of an Einstein-Montefiore complex which accounts for over 3,000 hospital beds.

Two other large general care systems are not attached to this complex. Misericordia staffs Fordham Hospital under an affiliation contract with the city. Together they have a bed complement of nearly 750. The other sizable institution is the Bronx-Lebanon Hospital Center, which resulted from the merger of the two voluntary hospitals in 1962. These three "systems" account for over 70 percent of the borough's nonfederal general care hospital beds. The remainder are dispersed among the relatively small and autonomous proprietary hospitals and the other voluntary institutions. In brief, the Bronx still has numerous independent institutions, but five of the largest hospitals in the area are affiliated either directly or indirectly with a medical school (see Table 8.1).

HOW THE COMPLEX GREW

The most significant point about the centralization which exists is that it is not the result of the implementation of any long-range plan. Rather, regionalization in the Bronx is a product of an ironic mixture of environmental circumstance, financial considerations, personal attitudes, and institutional interests, all of which are largely the unanticipated consequences of actions taken for other purposes.

An important environmental factor has been the simple fact that there is only one medical school in the borough. In areas where more than one medical school is located, institutional competition and rivalry seem to prevent comprehensive cooperative arrangements. Thus, Manhattan, with four medical schools, has not developed nearly the integration of facilities which has taken place in the Bronx. Similar difficulties have plagued the New York Regional Medical Program.[2] This federally supported program attempts to

TABLE 8.1

Bronx Hospitals, 1969

Map Number	Name	Bed Complement Total	General Care	Occupancy Rate
	Einstein-Montefiore Complex	3,033	2,349	
1.	Main Division, Montefiore Hospital	778	580	101.8
2.	Morrisania Hospital	331	331	84.7
3.	Einstein Division, Montefiore Hospital	366	321	82.9
4.	Bronx Municipal Hospital Center	1,208	767	75.1
5.	Lincoln Hospital	350	350	78.4
6.	Bronx State Hospital	1,015		92.1
7.	Bronx-Lebanon Hospital Center	564	564	91.8
	Misericordia-Fordham	733	733	
8.	Misericordia Hospital	332	332	94.4
9.	Fordham Hospital	401	401	82.6
	Other voluntary general hospitals	660	430	
10.	Bronx Eye Infirmary	44	44	60.1
11.	St. Barnabas Hospital	415	185	40.8
12.	Union Hospital	201	201	78.8
	Voluntary long-term hospitals	697		
13.	Calvary	109		98.0
14.	Daughters of Jacob	300		99.1
15.	Jewish Home and Hospital	288		97.4
	Proprietary hospitals	1,036	1,036	
16.	Mt. Eden	111	111	92.0
17.	Parkchester	208	208	88.6
18.	Pelham Bay	184	184	90.9
19.	Prospect	168	168	83.0
20.	Royal	91	91	74.7
21.	University Heights	50	50	75.8
22.	Westchester Square	224	224	83.9
23.	Veterans Administration Hospital	1,184	930	83.4

Note: Occupancy rates are for general care beds only, except for long-term hospitals and Bronx State Hospital. All rates are for the year 1968. All data are as reported by the Health and Hospital Planning Council.

coordinate the efforts of all six medical schools in the metropolitan area. The group has been able to approve very few projects since its inception and it appears that its progress will be minimal until tacit agreements are made to subdivide the region into smaller areas with one or two schools responsible for each area.

The inhibitory effects of competition among medical schools are further illustrated by the fact that even within the Bronx the possibility of another medical school delayed the movement toward centralization. Einstein-Montefiore could not have been considered a hyphenated complex for a considerable period of time. Part of the reason for this delay was Montefiore's desire to develop its own medical school. Discussions were carried on among Mount Sinai Hospital, Montefiore, and representatives of the Federation of Jewish Philanthropies, a fund-raising agency which would have been responsible for supplying some of the capital funds for a new school. It was hoped that a medical school could be created to serve both hospitals. It was only after this plan was abandoned and Mount Sinai proceeded to build its own medical school that relationships developed which made the Einstein-Montefiore complex possible. One practical conclusion: regionalization is most likely to occur where regions are defined so as to include only one medical school. This situation will not guarantee progress, but it appears to be a necessary prerequisite.

The affiliation between Einstein College and Bronx Municipal Hospital Center also had nothing to do with a conscious plan for regionalization. Staffing municipal hospitals was emerging as a problem when the Commissioner of Hospitals suggested to a group planning the new medical school that they build on vacant land near the municipal hospital center under construction in the Bronx. The action was mutually advantageous since it provided staff for the new hospital at a minimum cost and offered the college a large patient population to use as a teaching resource with the costs of hospitalization borne by the city. Out of this mutual interest the municipal center and the medical college came to depend upon each other.

Nor was the initial affiliation between Einstein and Lincoln Hospital part of a regional plan. In 1958 the Pediatrics Department at

Lincoln had deteriorated to the extent that it was without a director and had only one visiting pediatrician on its active staff. Nonpediatricians were running the crowded pediatric clinic. It was then that, owing to personal and professional ties with other segments of the staff and a nascent sense of community concern, Einstein voluntarily assumed responsibility for Lincoln Hospital's pediatric department. In the early 1960s the college gradually extended its affiliation to other departments, with some costs being met by the city, and in 1966 it entered into a comprehensive contract for complete professional services.

The city's affiliation system, aimed at ensuring the availability of physicians in municipal hospitals and not directly concerned with regionalization, added additional linkages to those previously described. In 1962 Montefiore and Morrisania were linked and in 1964 a contract was arranged between Fordham and Misericordia.

These affiliations have had a significant impact on the Bronx because a large portion of the borough's beds are in municipal facilities. In the Bronx nearly 40 percent of the nonfederal general care beds are city-owned, while in Manhattan the figure is closer to 20 percent and in Brooklyn and Queens it is about 25 percent. Consequently, affiliating the municipal hospitals has meant bringing the resources of a teaching hospital into contact with four of every ten general care beds in the borough. For our purposes the important point is that these affiliations were not conceived as steps toward regionalization. For the municipal hospitals they were necessary measures in obtaining medical staff. To the teaching institutions they represented an opportunity to broaden their teaching resources, obtain a new source of income, and expand services to the community. Neither party was directly concerned with implementing a regional plan.

The fact that initially Einstein College relied exclusively on municipal facilities led to a series of events which can be considered steps toward regionalization if only in an indirect, unanticipated manner. Shortly after the school opened it was confronted with pressure from its faculty for beds for their private patients. At that time, Einstein had no affiliation with Montefiore, nor could it establish one with another prestigious voluntary hospital. In order to meet the demand for private beds the school undertook to build its own hospital. While the hospital was being built the changes described earlier in the relations between Einstein and Montefiore took place. When the college hospital turned out to be too small, and when it experienced management troubles and was running at a deficit, a merger was arranged with Montefiore. The financial importance of this merger can be seen in the changes in the reimbursement rates under Blue Cross, Medicare, and Medicaid. After the hospital was placed under the administrative control of Montefiore, the two units were considered as one and Einstein became subject to a reimbursement rate equivalent to that of Montefiore. This resulted in an increase in income of about $25 per patient day. Thus an institution that was built to meet the faculty's insistence on private facilities was merged with another hospital largely for financial reasons. Neither the construction of the hospital nor the merger was undertaken as a step toward regionalization.

It is important to note that the single medical school in the Bronx has relied heavily on public resources for its development. Its site was made available through the recommendations of municipal officials. It utilizes a large municipal hospital as its primary teaching facility, and it receives a considerable portion of its revenues from diverse governmental sources. During the fiscal year 1967, Einstein received over $17.6 million in grants from the Department of Health, Education, and Welfare, more money than any other medical school in the nation save one.[3] It is probable that at least a portion of the salary of nearly every faculty member has been paid from a federal grant. This ability of the school to draw upon public resources was a source of strength until recently, when public funds available for medical research and training failed to expand and then actually began to decline.

An early effort at merger—but not necessarily at broadening community-wide services—was fostered by private philanthropy despite its declining capacity to cope with the vastly increasing needs of its member hospitals. Two key institutions in the Bronx, Montefiore and Bronx-Lebanon, are members of the Federation of Jewish Philanthropies. These institutions were founded to provide services for Jewish patients and opportunities for Jewish doctors. A 1961 study undertaken for the Federation[4] used these goals as guidelines for policy. The authors observed the demographic changes in the borough and recommended the eventual merger of Bronx, Lebanon, and Montefiore hospitals to form a "Bronx Jewish Hospital Center" at the Montefiore site, where services would be more easily accessible to Jews. The center was to have a strong affiliation with Einstein. Initially this plan appeared desirable although it proved difficult to carry through. Bronx and Lebanon merged and relations between Montefiore and Einstein grew closer. However, the union of Bronx-Lebanon with Montefiore has not taken place and it does not appear to be a likely prospect in the immediate future.

Some reasons can be suggested for the failure of this plan to move Bronx-Lebanon and merge it with Montefiore. Montefiore itself is reluctant to undertake an extensive affiliation with Bronx-Lebanon unless considerable additional resources are devoted to extensive capital development in order to make the hospital useful as a teaching institution for Einstein. Although the Federation might have exerted strong influence earlier to bring about such a merger, both its motivation and its ability to push the plan have waned. First, the declining role of philanthropy in hospital financing has permitted affiliated institutions to operate with greater autonomy. Income from the Federation provided less than 5 percent of its member hospitals' operating revenues in 1966 compared with almost 30 percent in the early 1940s and about 10 percent in the late 1950s. Second, conditions have changed and the need for institutions designed specifically to serve Jewish patients and physicians has diminished. Jewish doctors now encounter much less discrimination in obtaining hospital appointments and approximately three out of four Jewish patients do not seek care in a Federation hospital. At the same time the rapidly growing minority groups in the Bronx have come to rely upon the resources of these institutions. In 1960 the population of the Bronx was about 25 percent Negro and Puerto Rican; by 1966 the figure was almost 40 percent and it may reach 50 percent in 1970. The municipal hospitals staffed through affiliations with Jewish institutions serve an almost exclusively Negro and Puerto Rican population. A 1965 study found that 93 percent of the patients using the outpatient departments at Morrisania and Lincoln Hospitals were Negro or Puerto Rican.[5] This new reality has led to a new rationale for philanthropy: Jewish contributions are now directed toward helping the general community. Thus, while philanthropy contributed initially toward regionalization, its subsequent diminishing role in hospital financing has reduced its influence. Moreover, the regionalization pursued by the Federation was focused primarily on a consolidation of institutions under Jewish auspices rather than on an effort to rationalize community-wide services.

The actions of the Catholic Church, as well as those of Jewish organizations, have been influential in shaping the existing pattern of health care in the Bronx. The closing of St. Francis Hospital in 1966 placed almost the entire responsibility for health services in the South Bronx on Lincoln Hospital. In the short run the effect has probably been to overburden an aged facility. In the long run the effect will probably be a more rational arrangement. The design of the new Lincoln Hospital, which is to be built on a site near St. Francis, includes a bed capacity larger than the combined total of the existing Lincoln and the former St. Francis hospitals. Since over 70 percent of St. Francis's patients were ward patients, most of whose care was paid for by the city, the hospital was probably serving a population not much different from that cared for in a municipal institution. The physical plant of St. Francis was deteriorating. To rebuild it on the same site in proximity to a municipal hospital intended to serve the same population would have been wasteful duplication.

Other criticisms can be and have been made about the closing of St. Francis.[6] There was inadequate planning for the period which will elapse before the new Lincoln Hospital becomes operational. Given the pace of municipal construction, this could mean a decade. Decisions affecting the health status of an entire community were made with little public discussion, largely by persons who were unaccountable to residents of the neighborhood. Whether or not it was their intention, the long-range effect of the closing of St. Francis will be to facilitate regionalization.

The Catholic Church's other important center in the Bronx is Misericordia Hospital, which in 1964 entered into an affiliation contract with Fordham Hospital to help provide services to the neighborhoods of both hospitals. Howard Brown, a non-Catholic, the former New York City Health Services Administrator, was hired to direct the program of ambulatory services. The Misericordia-Fordham complex is seeking an affiliation with Einstein. However, the college, which is already committed to two municipal hospitals and affiliated with Montefiore, is reluctant to extend itself further. Misericordia faces an uncertain future. To maintain itself as a reputable institution it feels obliged to affiliate with a medical college, but if Einstein does not agree, the hospital will be in a difficult position, although the future relocation of New York Medical College in Westchester may provide new opportunities.

The final factor which helps to explain the nature of the Bronx hospital system is the personality and actions of Dr. Martin Cherkasky. As director of Montefiore Hospital, he has demonstrated a commitment to making his hospital a center of progressive medical care. He supported prepaid group practice and from 1948 to 1969 Montefiore housed an HIP group which enjoyed an excellent reputation. He was influential in developing the city's affiliation system and Montefiore was one of the first voluntary hospitals to affiliate with a municipal institution. The present contract is most extensive and embraces almost all services including nursing. As an outgrowth of this relationship Montefiore has sponsored an OEO-financed neighborhood health center in Morrisania's area. The leadership provided by Cherkasky and the attention he has drawn to his hospital's many innovative programs have contributed to much of the progress that the Bronx has made in medical matters.

WHY THE COMPLEX IS NOT LARGER

So far we have pointed out that the integration in health care in the Bronx has not been an outgrowth of a conscious effort to implement a regional plan. Interhospital relationships have been explained by a unique combination of chance, personal drive, financial considerations, and a variety of other institutional and interest group concerns. As important as why some integration has occurred is why the process has not gone further.

Two general constraints prevented the growth of a comprehensive university-centered medical complex. One has been the reluctance of independent institutions to relinquish their autonomy or to restrict their activities in the interest of more efficient joint operations. The other is the reluctance of the crucial central elements, the medical school and its principal teaching hospital, to extend their resources beyond limited areas for fear that further expansion would weaken their capacity to provide proper teaching opportunities and experiences.

Both constraints have operated in the Bronx. We have previously mentioned the teaching institutions' reluctance to extend themselves and perhaps to lower the caliber of their services. That Bronx-Lebanon and Montefiore did not merge partially reflected this concern. The difficulty in establishing an affiliation between Misericordia and Einstein has a similar background. Consequently, many of the area's hospitals remain outside the central complex.

There are also pressures for autonomy in the Bronx. One important source of pressure is the independent private practitioner. The proprietary hospitals, with which many private physicians are associated, account for a large portion of the borough's hospital beds. One of every five general care beds in the Bronx is in a proprietary hospital. The implications are twofold. First, because of this non-academic orientation, financial interests, and the ideology of the owners, these hospitals will remain outside of any regional complex. The relationships which may develop between the profit and the not-for-profit sectors are in the use of central laboratories and interchange of medical records. Second, it is possible to state that a large proprietary sector indirectly contributes to the integration that does exist. It has provided physicians whose philosophy of medical practice differs from those at the hub of the medical school with a broad domain in which to function. Expansion of the school's activities has taken place without impinging on their practices. Consequently, the town-gown conflicts have not been as severe as they might have been.

The majority of private practitioners in the Bronx have remained isolated from the Einstein-Montefiore complex. These doctors and the school have proceeded on the theory that they have nothing to do with each other. Only a few members of the County Medical Society are affiliated with either Einstein or Montefiore. The active members feel alienated from most of the developments in the Bronx and decry their lack of influence. In this respect, their attitude is similar to that of their patients who bemoan the fact that they have no control over the available health services. These attitudes were reflected in the support that the Society gave Borough President Herman Badillo and the local residents in their pressure to keep St. Francis open. The private practitioners disliked the prospect of a local hospital closing its doors and in the process enhancing the role of the municipal hospitals, Montefiore, and Einstein.

Elected officials have had a relatively minor role in shaping the development of hospital services in the Bronx. Their participation is sporadic, elicited by dramatic issues. A frequent concern is with projects included in or excluded from the capital budget. New structures represent concrete accomplishments for which officials can take credit. Moreover, the Board of Estimate must approve the capital budget and the informal rules under which the Board operates give each borough president considerable influence over projects in his area. Thus, finding a site for, and speeding the construction of, a new Lincoln Hospital was a political objective of Borough President Badillo.

The recent legislation authorizing the establishment of an independent corporation to manage municipal hospitals attracted the attention of local officials. The City Council held public hearings on the bill. Borough President Badillo, State Senator Robert Garcia, and other political figures objected to the proposed corporation because they felt it would not be responsive to the public's needs. Suggestions for improving public accountability included retaining hospital management as a function of the Department of Hospitals and adding the statutory requirement that each hospital have an advisory board composed of local residents. Modifications in the legislation in accordance with the latter suggestion were made, so it appears that the politicians have been effective in this regard. However, their relations to hospital affairs have been limited to dramatic issues like capital projects and the reorganization of municipal agencies.

THE MODEL, THE EXISTING SYSTEM, AND THE FUTURE

While the existing hospital system or systems in the Bronx have not resulted from a conscious effort to implement a regional plan, they can be evaluated in terms of such a model. Five criticisms can be made of the present arrangement. First, cooperation among institutions in the Bronx, while more advanced than in other regions, is still not near optimal levels. The coordination of activities and the sharing of resources are limited to the medical school, Montefiore Hospital, and their affiliates. The other hospitals, which provide more than half the total days of care in the borough, remain unrelated to the complex. Patients at the proprietary and smaller voluntary institutions are unable to avail themselves of the skill and knowledge concentrated at "the well-spring of medical science represented in the teaching hospital and medical school." In brief, there is a need for the teaching institutions to open their services to a broader segment of the hospital system in the Bronx.

Second, there is an uneven distribution of facilities within the borough. The newer and larger facilities are located in the northern part of the borough while the southern part has a large population with unmet needs. Surveys and studies indicate that poverty and morbidity are highly correlated and it is in the south where the poor are heavily concentrated. Yet this area has the oldest hospitals. The main building of Lincoln Hospital was erected in the 1890s and little renovation or expansion has taken place since the 1930s. Ten years ago the Health and Hospital Planning Council reported that it was impractical and uneconomical to modernize the hospital.[7] Rebuilding it may properly be deemed urgent. In addition, the supply of hospital beds in the south has been shrinking while the population continues to expand. The closing of St. Francis Hospital reduced the inadequate total by over 300 beds. The plans for Morrisania Hospital reinforce this trend: originally Morrisania, in the South Bronx, was to be closed upon the completion of a new municipal hospital which was to be built adjacent to Montefiore in the north. The closing of Morrisania was subsequently left pending until the completion of the new hospital; by now it has been reaffirmed. While the need is greatest in the south and public pressure is increasingly for decentralized or community-oriented facilities, health and hospital services continue to be concentrated and expanded in the northern portions of the Bronx.

The Bronx, like all of New York City, needs improved ambulatory services. As indicated elsewhere in this volume, the hospital outpatient department and particularly the emergency room now serve as a primary source of medical care for the urban poor. New demands are acutely manifest at the municipal hospitals in the Bronx (see Table 8.2). For example, emergency visits at Lincoln Hospital climbed from 101,226 in 1961 to 185,527 in 1967. At Morrisania the same time period witnessed a rise from 61,765 to 134,083 emergency room visits. While these developments represent the continuing *ad hoc* adaptation by hospitals to these new demands, it is certainly now not considered ideal. The regional system envisioned by the Piel Commission would include an expanded network of ambulatory care facilities to meet the public's needs.

Some measures to improve the system have been taken. In an effort to deal effectively with the increasing patient load at its affiliated institution, Montefiore Hospital has sponsored a Neighborhood Medical Care Demonstration project,[8] now known as the Martin Luther King, Jr. Neighborhood Health Center. With financial support from the Office of Economic Opportunity, an ambulatory center has been built and staffed to serve a population of about 45,000 in the Morrisania and Tremont health districts. The center is organized around medical teams who provide continuous care for entire families. While these changes are undoubtedly valuable, they have proved to be expensive. In 1968 the center served approximately 4,000 families at a cost of about $4.8 million.

The need for qualitative and quantitative changes in the capacity for ambulatory care, the high cost of such changes, and decreased financial support for this care owing to restrictions in insurance and welfare programs confront the medical system in the Bronx with additional problems.

Implicit in the concept of a regional system is the assumption that coordination of services will result in a less costly operation. It is anticipated that specialized treatment and equipment would be concentrated in the central university hospital with correspondingly high cost. However, routine services and treatment are to be performed at the community hospitals where costs could be lower. In the Bronx, hospital relationships have not always been characterized by functional differentiation. The pattern has been an upgrading

TABLE 8.2

Ambulatory Visits to Bronx Hospitals, 1967

	Total	Outpatient Department	Emergency Room
Montefiore Hospital	106,457	78,590	27,867
Morrisania Hospital	207,041	135,958	134,083
Montefiore Neighborhood Medical Care Demonstration	14,630	n.a.	n.a.
Bronx Municipal Center	394,501*	268,452	126,049
Lincoln Hospital	383,210*	197,683	185,527
Bronx-Lebanon Hospital	153,442*	103,800	49,642
Bronx-Lebanon Morrisania Center	14,743	n.a.	n.a.
Misericordia Hospital	46,198	25,399	20,799
Fordham Hospital	211,142	123,767	87,375
St. Barnabas Hospital	6,540	6,371	169
Bronx Eye Infirmary	23,892	20,619	3,273
Union Hospital	612	612	
All proprietary hospitals	7,866	7,866	n.a.

Source: Health and Hospital Planning Council.
n.a. = Not available.
* Includes visits to free-standing clinic.

of nonuniversity hospitals with corresponding increases in costs. Affiliation contracts for municipal general hospitals have been more costly than anticipated. In addition, routine nonspecialized services at the central institutions are expensive. According to the most recent Medicaid figures, a clinic visit to Montefiore Hospital costs over thirty dollars![9] The leaders of the complex have not been adequately concerned with restraining cost increases.

Finally, hospitals have not met the problems presented by demands for community participation in decisions involving health services. Conflicts over the role of consumers have surfaced. In New York City the establishment of a comprehensive health planning body was stalemated for over two years because of the requirement that a place be made for consumer representatives. The role of local residents was a troublesome issue in the design of the new hospital corporation. The Lincoln Hospital Mental Health Center was the focus of a battle over the role of local residents and nonprofessional personnel in policy-making.

Several factors have given weight to the desire for broad participation in health and hospital decision-making. The "private" hospitals in New York City receive from tax funds about $125 million annually for the care of the indigent and medically indigent. An additional $140 million is paid to many of the same institutions by the city through its affiliation contracts. According to a 1967 census of hospital patients in southern New York, the care of over 30 percent of the patients in voluntary hospitals is paid for by federal Medicare dollars. These shifts in financing have been accompanied by changes in citizens' attitudes toward medical care. Since a substantial portion of all hospital care, regardless of whether in a municipal, voluntary, or proprietary facility, is financed by public funds and practically all care is reimbursed through some third-party mechanism, it is felt that hospitals should be viewed more as public utilities than as private enterprises or charitable operations. Medical care is increasingly assuming the quality of a public service similar to education in the public's mind. Access to care is considered a right rather than a privilege and to ensure this right it is argued that representatives of the consumer public should exercise some control over the institutions.

Those who are reluctant to institute extensive changes have their reasons. They claim that planning for and provision of health services require expertise which is more likely to characterize doctors and hospital administrators than local residents. Ignoring expertise is likely to lead to low quality and inefficiency in the delivery of care. In addition, the mission of educational institutions is not solely, or even primarily, that of providing services to local residents. Medical schools train doctors for the entire nation and are engaged in the search for new knowledge. Most of the federal money which they receive is spent to further these goals and and not to provide services. They can meet the objectives only if they meet the standards of scientific inquiry and professional education.

It is not easy to define roles for physicians, administrators, para-professionals, and local residents in health and hospital decision-making. The problem may be especially difficult in the Bronx because of the differences between the leaders of a heavily Jewish medical complex and a patient population which has a large proportion of Negroes and Puerto Ricans. The leaders of the important institutions in the Bronx will undoubtedly face continuing pressure for greater participation from the community. So far they have not fully met this challenge.

The future development of a regional system in the Bronx can also be discussed in terms of paths which it may take that depart from the planners' model. First, from the point of view of regionalization, it would be desirable for the interrelationships among existing institutions to be expanded. Affiliations between Bronx-Lebanon and Montefiore and between Einstein and Misericordia might be desirable. Yet these steps are not likely to take place. The school's present ties include one voluntary and two municipal hospitals. Teaching members of the faculty feel that further commitments would reduce their capacity to maintain a high-quality teaching program.

Present hospital planning includes measures to relieve the uneven distribution of facilities. The city's capital budget already provides for a new enlarged Lincoln Hospital to be built at 149th Street and Park Avenue. It is considered a priority project and the State Health and Mental Hygiene Facilities Improvement Corporation has scheduled its construction. The capital budget also authorizes the replacement of Fordham Hospital in the same area in which it is presently located. These projects will help maintain a degree of accessibility to inpatient care in the communities concerned. Another item in the capital budget is a new North Central Bronx Hospital to be built adjacent to Montefiore. As noted above, this project was originally designed as a replacement for Morrisania. Subsequently, the structure was designated as a new hospital and the future of Morrisania was reconsidered. It has now been decided to phase out the hospital and convert Morrisania to a comprehensive ambulatory care facility. The plans for Lincoln and Fordham hospitals provide an opportunity to improve the geographic distribution of hospital beds.

The future of consumer participation in the formulation of health services policy remains moot. The proper role for the community has not been clearly defined. The legislation creating the Health and Hospitals Corporation requires that advisory boards of members representative of the community served be established for each hospital. In accord with guidelines set by the OEO, Montefiore Hospital has a community advisory board for its demonstration project. Such bodies might also be established for voluntary hospitals. In some contexts it may prove desirable and practical to give representatives more than merely an advisory role. Moreover, legislation now recognizes a role for consumers and it is likely that this trend will continue.

Plans for meeting ambulatory care needs have centered on a network of neighborhood family care centers (NFCCs) to be built by the city. If current commitments are met, the following ambulatory facilities will be constructed in the Bronx: a health center at the new North Central Bronx Hospital, a health center at the new Lincoln Hospital, an NFCC in the vicinity of Fordham Hospital, an NFCC at the site of St. Francis Hospital, expanded ambulatory services at the Tremont district health center, an NFCC at Morrisania Hospital, and NFCCs in the Hunts Point and Soundview areas (see Table 8.3).

Several points should be made about these plans for increased ambulatory services. First, the way in which they are operated and their relationship to municipal hospitals and their affiliates will de-

TABLE 8.3

1969–1970 Capital Budget, Health Services Administration, Projects in the Bronx[a]

Description	Estimated Total Cost	Authorizations Current	Authorizations Prior	Prior Expenditures
North Central Bronx Hospital	$42,169,700	$ 150,000	$1,322,000	$ 857,736
Replace Fordham Hospital	32,000,000	1,400,000	225,000	
Replace Lincoln Hospital[b]	74,452,000		7,085,000	2,261,153
NFCC near present Fordham Hospital[b]	5,911,000	288,000	177,000	
St. Francis NFCC[b]	4,131,000	3,429,000	230,000	143,022
Ambulatory services at Tremont Health Center	1,660,000	100,000	265,400	
Hunts Point NFCC[b]	5,000,000			
Convert St. Francis Hospital to ambulatory center	3,000,000		3,000,000	
NFCC at Morrisania Hospital	4,135,000		215,000	
Soundview NFCC	4,150,000		230,000	
Crotona Park–Highbridge Mental Health Center	15,750,000	[c]	1,000,000	

Source: City of New York, *Capital Budget, 1969–70*.
[a] Excludes some authorizations for renovations and alterations.
[b] Includes community mental health unit.
[c] Included in a lump-sum site acquisition authorization.

termine the extent to which they conform to a regional model. In the theory of regionalization each ambulatory facility is assigned a back-up hospital which is expected to make available when necessary specialized manpower, facilities, and equipment. This is the intended arrangement for the network of structures which the city expects to construct. However, this intention is not made explicit in the legislation creating the Health and Hospitals Corporation. While the statute specified July 1, 1970, as the date when the corporation would assume responsibility for operating municipal hospitals and committed a minimum specified amount, $175 million, of city funds for this purpose, it made no similar provision for ambulatory facilities. The law only stated that "within a reasonable time" responsibility for other than hospital facilities should be transferred to the corporation. Moreover, there was no guarantee of financial support from the city for nonhospital facilities.

Securing operating funds for multiple ambulatory centers is likely to prove exceedingly difficult. Plans for these facilities were formulated when Medicaid eligibility requirements and payments were much more liberal than now. Consequently, state and federal support for ambulatory services will not be as extensive as originally anticipated. Moreover, given the fiscal problems facing New York City, it is questionable whether local tax funds will be available to support the complete network of facilities which the capital budget authorizes.

The interesting lesson to be extracted from progress made in the Bronx toward "regionalization" is that the reforms did not flow from a predetermined commitment to move in this direction or to an articulated design to guide such movement. Rather, the progress that was made in solving a series of specific challenges resulted in a more rational design. The transformations are the product of a set of circumstances not likely to be duplicated in other areas. The limited achievements in the Bronx required a strong institution with expansionary management, command over considerable resources, and influence within a medical school; other institutions compelled by manpower shortages, financial difficulties, and/or deteriorating physical plant to sacrifice their autonomy or even their existence; and a minority population which up to now has been poorly organized and consequently unable to utilize the leverage inherent in their growing numbers. The near impossibility and the questionable desirability of re-creating these conditions in other localities, coupled with the limited gains they have made possible, indicate that the implementation of regional designs will remain a difficult process.

9
TB CONTROL

THE ERADICATION of tuberculosis suddenly burst into the realm of possibility with the introduction in 1952 of potent specific antibiotics, chiefly isoniazid, para-aminosalycilic acid, and streptomycin, all of which have both therapeutic and prophylactic properties. There followed a precipitous decline in the census of active cases; epidemiologic projections were altered; and it was confidently assumed that tuberculosis would no longer constitute a serious problem. Actually, however, events have been less felicitous: impressive technologic capability (epidemiologists assert that the drugs are potentially effective in over 95 percent of newly diagnosed cases) has been limited by countervailing pathogens which maintain the disease incidence at a stubborn level, and though existent health structures have adapted intensively to the new therapy, more apposite structures and manpower for its optimal implementation have not been developed. The interaction of changing technology, social forces, and institutional medicine, and their impact upon tuberculosis control of the past fifteen years in New York City, constitute an instructive case history with implications for current urban health planning.

SOME BACKGROUND FACTS ABOUT TUBERCULOSIS AND TUBERCULOSIS CONTROL

Classically, a case study starts with a history of its subject. Tuberculosis, recognized as a disease entity for centuries, increased in prevalence and virulence to become one of the worst side effects of the industrial revolution and the attendant urbanization, so that by the beginning of this century it was the chief cause of death in the

United States. Following isolation of the pathogen, the tubercle bacillus, considerable progress began to be made in tuberculosis control through the development within a few years of tuberculin testing and roentgenology for early diagnosis, and through the discovery of an effective therapeutic technique in complete bed rest and good nursing. Subsequently, bold techniques of surgical intervention were devised for selected patients, superimposed upon but not replacing the long-term bed care. In the absence of any immunizing agent or procedure, lengthy isolation of the patient with active tuberculosis constituted the only effective prophylaxis for the community.

In the past, two characteristics have been responsible for the extraordinary stubbornness of tuberculosis, exceeding that of any other major infectious disease: the almost indefinite persistence of the dormant pathogen within the host (it is estimated that even today as much as 25 percent of the total population in the United States may be infected, though in very few will the disease become active), and the failure of many patients to recover completely from active infection and to acquire subsequent immunity; in fact, the recovered patient was always at high risk of subsequent reactivation. Accordingly, in the pre-chemotherapeutic years, tuberculosis control proceeded along two main axes: provision of a sufficient number of beds for long-term hospitalization and vigorous case-finding for early identification and isolation of patients with active disease.

The actual scale of the disease and the dramatic gain in control are reflected in the annual morbidity and mortality statistics published by the New York City Department of Health (Table 9.1). By 1950, the tuberculosis new case rate (83 per 100,000) represented a reduction of 80 percent from its 1900–1904 level of 400 per 100,000; mortality declined still more impressively over the same time span from 220 to 27 per 100,000. To a considerable extent, these gains had been effected as a result of environmental and social improvements: specific public health measures, industrial legislation, enhanced standard of living. Awareness of essential limitations in medical control over the disease served to maintain apprehensive, tentative attitudes toward its occurrence and treatment, evident in the paradoxical situation of the 1940s when, in marked contrast

TABLE 9.1

Changing Dimensions of Tuberculosis in New York City, 1900–1966

Year[a]	New Cases[b]		Deaths		Deaths per 100 New Cases Reported
	No.	Rate (per 100,000)	No.	Rate (per 100,000)	
1900–4	14,500	396	8,100	220	56
1910–14	24,700	498	8,700	176	35
1920–24	12,700	214	5,200	88	41
1930–34	10,800	154	4,150	59	38
1940–44	8,300	109	3,300	44	40
1950	6,518	83	2,150	27	33
1953	6,110	78	1,180	15	19
1955	5,060	65	1,025	13	20
1960	3,900	50	760	9.8	19
1961	3,635	47	690	8.8	19
1962	3,700	48	695	8.9	19
1963	4,060	52	645	8.3	16
1964	3,380	43	535	6.8	16
1965	3,390	43	550	6.9	16
1966	2,950	37	500	6.2	17

Source: Department of Health, City of New York.
[a] For the years 1900 to 1944, the figures represent a quinquennial average.
[b] Excludes primary tuberculosis (children under ten years).

to declining new case rates, tuberculosis inpatient populations increased continuously, particularly in the municipal hospitals where bed complement for the patients rose by a third and average occupancy rates persisted at 99 percent; similar utilization trends were seen in the far smaller nonpublic sector.

Into this escalating hospital- or sanatorium-based program of tuberculosis care was imposed in 1952 the radically new chemotherapy whose action was to terminate rapidly—within a matter of weeks or at most several months, dependent upon severity—the acute infectious phase of the disease and to permit discharge of the patient to the community for continued treatment at home in ambulatory status under medical supervision.

The *modus operandi* of chemotherapy is to destroy the active pathogen; since the tubercle bacillus multiplies slowly and can remain dormant for a period of years, vigorous drug therapy must continue uninterrupted long after the disease has passed the communicable phase. Of even greater potential significance is the prophylactic action of chemotherapy in infected individuals under the risk of developing *active* tuberculosis.

The clinical effect of chemotherapy has been to transform treatment of tuberculosis from primarily passive long-term hospital care of patients with active symptomatic disease to vigorous drug intervention with patients in the active or arrested phases of the disease and, more recently, with infected individuals to avoid the development of active disease. Except for the communicable phase of the active disease, hospitalization is neither required nor desirable. Close and restrictive patient supervision is not indicated; isolation, vocational retraining, and basic rehabilitation are scientific anachronisms.

The impact of chemotherapy upon the requirement for hospital beds was prompt and unequivocal: in the summer of 1953, the upward trend in the tuberculosis inpatient caseload of the New York hospitals was reversed for the first time, and the decline continued dramatically, producing within five years a net loss of well over 30 percent in beds and of almost 45 percent in annual patient-days.[1] By 1968 the city bed capacity had been lowered to under 1,500, of which only 26 are in voluntary hospitals. This is in dramatic contrast to an estimated future requirement of 9,000 made about twenty years ago (1948).[2] Current recommendations are for further reductions at the rate of 100 beds annually, over the next five-year period.[3] In terms of health policy and planning, emphasis has been shifting from facilities expansion, improved financing for long-term care, and mass diagnostic X-ray services to preventive and therapeutic outpatient services and the concentration of control efforts upon specific high-risk populations.

Nationwide, no less than in the city, a spectacular reduction occurred in the amount of active disease following the introduction of chemotherapy. This was reflected in an annual decrease in new cases, averaging over 6 percent in the years between 1953 and 1959, decelerating sharply in 1960, and reaching a standstill in 1961–63. In New York City, 1962 actually saw a reversal in trend with a rise in the new case rate. This unanticipated stubbornness rearoused public health concern and was reflected in numerous studies on national and local levels aimed at identifying realistic program priorities. Chief among these was the U.S. Surgeon General's Task Force on Tuberculosis Control which recommended in 1963 federal grants to the states for the implementation of an intensive nationwide prophylactic program, which might be expected in ten years to reduce new case incidence by 60 percent, as opposed to an anticipated 30 percent if current trends were to continue.

In New York City, even while the trend of new cases was sharply downward, various standing and *ad hoc* committees called attention to serious shortcomings of personnel, particularly in the municipal hospital system, and the lack of effective coordination between inpatient and ambulatory services. In addition, these committees called attention to the need for more effective preventive measures based primarily upon intensified early case-finding and secondary prevention through vigorous treatment of incompletely recovered patients. The Ramapo Conference (1961) explored in detail the socioeconomic deterrents to effective treatment of the deprived population among whom infection is increasingly concentrated. Reviewing a decade of experience with isoniazid treatment, the New York City Department of Health found in 1962 that tuberculosis had become less frequent (annual new case decline of 40 percent), less fatal (over 50 percent reduction in annual deaths), and increasingly concentrated within specific geographic areas of the city (the ghettos) and among the lowest-income segments of the population (the aged and minorities). It concluded: "During the next decade a massive assault must be directed against the real root of the disease which is poverty, if substantial progress toward its eradication is to be made." This conclusion was in substantial agreement with national findings of the Surgeon General's Task Force of the following year, which emphasized the concentration of the disease in specific urban centers and its disproportionate prevalence among nonwhites.

The problem of imperfect adaptation to a revolutionized medical technology in New York City's program of tuberculosis control can be approached by stipulating a standard, say, the recommendations of the Ramapo Conference (1961), which addressed itself to specific comprehensive problems—the prevention of exogenous infection, more effective case-finding, inadequacies in treatment, and social deterrents to effective utilization of services—and investigating the response to the recommendations advanced in the report. Another reference point, perhaps more cogent because of its technical specificity, would be the Report of the Surgeon General's Task Force. Given a highly specific set of priorities, clearly applicable to New York City, one could explore to what extent these have been implemented, and what has determined the selection or rejection of specific recommendations.

The most recent survey of the city's tuberculosis control effort is summarized in the Report of the Task Force on Tuberculosis in New York City, December, 1968, which undertook a review for the purpose of producing a suitable medium-range (five-year) program for integration with comprehensive health planning that might be undertaken by the city in compliance with Public Law 89-749, a precondition for qualifying for federal health funds.

A few key indices will help to clarify trends in tuberculosis in New York City over the past decade (see Table 9.2). The startling disparity between the city and the nation is not distinctive to New

TABLE 9.2

New Active Tuberculosis Case Rate, New York City and the Nation,
1955–1967

	1955–57 average (per 100,000)	1965–67 average (per 100,000)
United States	42.2	24.2
New York City	78.7	47.7
Manhattan	163.7	84.7
Bronx	59.7	42.3
Brooklyn	62.0	47.0
Queens	35.7	23.3
Richmond	36.0	22.0

New Active Tuberculosis Cases by Ethnic Group, New York City,
1965–1967

	Average Number of New Cases	Average Annual Case Rate	Percent of Total Cases
Nonwhite	1,631	116.6	48.2
Puerto Rican	382	50.9	11.3
Other Whites	1,371	23.9	40.5

York. In 1965 New York City was outranked in new case rates by at least seven other cities, each characterized by a large nonwhite population: Newark, Baltimore, San Francisco, Detroit, Washington, D.C., Chicago, and Jersey City. County-based statistics may also obscure heavy disease concentration in several other urban centers, such as Miami. Nevertheless, New York's extraordinary size yields a total caseload impressive in sheer numbers: 3,542 (1967), 8 percent of a national total of just under 45,500. The city's total is exceeded by only two states—New York (obviously) and California. It must further be recalled that the city's average is heavily determined by the rate for Manhattan, which contains the extremes in neighborhood variation: Kips Bay and Yorkville with a rate of 22, almost the lowest in the city, and Central Harlem with a rate of 160, by far the highest.

The principal sources of recalcitrance found by the Task Force can be grouped as follows: functional problems of the municipal health services system, of which tuberculosis control is a (not especially favored or conspicuous) subset; resource problems of a residual specialty, interesting chiefly to epidemiologists and community medicine specialists and of only passing professional concern to clinicians; the lag between current scientific thought and current practice and belief—among professionals, institutions, paraprofessionals, patients, and the general public; the inextricability of public health aspects of tuberculosis from its socioeconomic dimensions; and the problem of delivering health services to the poor who are primarily nonwhite.

DIFFICULTIES OF CHANGE
IN THE PUBLIC SECTOR

For the obvious reasons of chronicity and contagion, tuberculosis control has long been a responsibility of the public sector, with some supplemental resources contributed by philanthropy. This was true throughout the pre-chemotherapeutic era when bed supply consistently fell short of patient need despite declining incidence. As late as 1948, the expansion of voluntary treatment facilities was recommended, particularly through the opening of general hospital beds to active tuberculosis patients. Additionally, after-care, rehabilitation, and social programs generally, to the extent that they were available, were provided by voluntary agencies. With the vast reduction in bed requirements starting in the 1950s, following the abandonment of isolation as critical to tuberculosis management, programmatic efforts became in effect a municipal monopoly. As of 1968, there were only 26 beds in the voluntary sector (20 in Montefiore; 6 in New York Hospital), and 1,425 in the municipal sector (somewhat over 8 percent of the total municipal hospital bed complement). As far as outpatient services are concerned, of 14,000 ambulatory patients under care in 1967 only 300 were treated by voluntary general hospitals. Since the role of the State of New York is almost exclusively financial, tuberculosis treatment services are a subsystem of the municipal health and hospital system, which is in turn a subsystem of New York's municipal government. No other area of personal medical service operates so completely within the municipal system, which makes it a paradigm of noncompetitive, nonsupplemented public service, in sharp contrast to other parts of the medical complex that operate under both governmental and nongovernmental control. Accordingly the characteristics of tuberculosis services are to a great extent reflective of the general and medical governmental systems.

STRUCTURE

Under the municipal umbrella, many authorities overlap in the production of tuberculosis services. The structure is essentially modular. Inpatient care is furnished by nine municipal hospitals, with about 85 percent of the total beds contained in four very large services, each of which operates completely independently with consequent wide variation in professional practices and standards and in administrative policy. This pattern has clearly negative implications for epidemiological control. Uniformity is absent even on such key matters as criteria for admission and discharge and for clinical management. Except for one small service in Staten Island (Seaview Hospital with about twenty-five beds), tuberculosis inpatient care has gradually been included under the affiliation contracts between the city and the medical schools and voluntary teaching hospitals for professional services. Outpatient services, that is, preventive and post-hospital, are provided by combined health-hospital clinics attached to seven hospital inpatient services, and a network of twenty-one free-standing district clinics dispersed throughout the city.

Communication lines within this system are highly attenuated; coordination between tuberculosis services and external health agencies offering general and specialized medical services as well as social agencies serving the tuberculous poor (welfare, housing, narcotics and alcohol control) is all but nonexistent. Within the tuberculosis system, specific essential services (patient nursing, laboratory services, public health nursing) also operate with a degree of autonomy and an absence of coordination that make for grave inefficiency in individual patient care, and, more significantly for this study, preclude effective implementation of any broad policy change that might be determined at the top.

RESOURCES

In common with all municipal health services, as emphasized by the Piel Report (1967), tuberculosis control suffers serious shortages of manpower, equipment, and funds. Professional manpower for inpatient services, now included in the affiliation contracts, has provided at least minimal medical services to the hospitalized for the last several years. But given the relative lack of interest of medical schools and voluntary hospitals in the disease, the city has not received any significant augmentation of professional staff and has had to rely largely on community practitioners who are available on a part-time basis and those who contract for a specific number of "sessions" per week, two groups that are likely to be a step or two behind current theory and practice. Nor have affiliation contracts provided the professional thrust for significant innovative approaches, with one impressive exception. Medical school affiliation by and large has reinforced, or at least not significantly attenuated, entrenched attitudes and practices. Supportive personnel within the hospital system, contractually the responsibility of the city, is conspicuously under-supplied and minimally trained. Here we have a special case of municipal health manpower where the city's generally unfavorable competitive position is aggravated by the threatening image of tuber-culosis in the unsophisticated labor market of health workers.

Rigidities that impede adjustments in wage schedules to meet the market and that preclude replacing anachronistic job slots with others more appropriate to current practice and shifting allocations from low-priority requirements to strengthen high-priority needs were specified by the Piel Report as deleterious to the system as a whole. But they are mortal to any program for change. In the case of tuberculosis, shifting requirements over the past decade may be inferred from Figure 9.1, which illustrates the unabated rise in total number of patients under treatment, from 9,000 (1959) to over 14,000 (1967), or a 55 percent increase within eight years. How-ever, this rise masks two contrasting trends: a precipitate increase of almost 125 percent in clinic patients, and a decline in the inpatient total to about 35 percent of its earlier level. Such a radical shift in requirements by different parts of the system underscores the need for flexibility in the use of manpower and other resources. An ex-panded and revitalized ambulatory service is clearly needed and at least part of the additional personnel could be obtained by transfers from the shrinking inpatient operations. But such transfers are ex-ceedingly difficult to engineer in the face of bureaucratic autonomy of the several parts of the system.

THE LAG BETWEEN THEORY
AND PRACTICE

Not subject to direct assessment but of unequivocal significance in the implementation of programmatic change have been the per-sistence of old attitudes and practices and the slow diffusion of new concepts at all levels. The characteristic lag between scientific leadership and patients, practitioners, and the public is particularly tenacious in the case of tuberculosis control. Many practitioners are loath to alter their long-held views about the nature of contagion and the desirability of prolonged bed rest. Both students and workers entering the medical field, particularly nurses, often assimilate these attitudes rather than those more congruent with advanced scientific knowledge. The lag on the part of the public is likewise an important impediment to the modification of therapy.

At the professional level, the average length of hospitalization

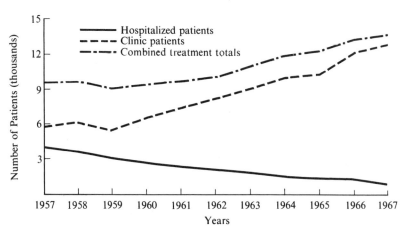

Figure 9.1. Changing Modes of Tuberculosis Treatment
in New York City, 1957-1967

ranges from two to three months to over a year, to a great extent reflecting variations in medical criteria for discharge. More importantly, city-wide average length of stay per medically approved discharge consistently exceeds the period of under six months currently recommended by epidemiologists to be adequate for the return of the patient to home or clinic care.

Subprofessional employees receive differential pay for employment on tuberculosis services, and not infrequently recovered tuberculosis patients experience difficulties in securing employment. Patients, their families, and the general public do not readily accept the current view that a history of tuberculosis does not disqualify an individual for active physical employment or require a radical shift toward a sedentary, restricted life-style.

HEALTH SERVICES IN THE PURVIEW OF
THE RACIAL REVOLUTION

Nonspecific to tuberculosis treatment and control programs but of direct consequence to their progress is the ongoing race revolution. In its struggle to gain power the black community has adopted the strategy of rejecting traditional services planned, directed, and produced by the white-dominated establishment. Health services have not constituted a key target in the same manner as have education and welfare. Direct action has been concentrated in efforts to unionize black and Puerto Rican health employees and to secure more equitable participation in the white-monopolized construction trades. Nevertheless, efforts of the recent past to introduce new structures (neighborhood health centers) and new programs (community mental health) have mobilized black opposition to professional leadership and have led to demands for active participation by representatives of the community at all levels—planning, policy determination, direction, management, preferential employment—as a condition for community acceptance. The 1968 Report of the Task Force on Tuberculosis in New York City found: "So strong is the resistance to having services improved by the 'establishment' that suggestions which are technically sound may be rejected, perhaps violently. These social trends are noted because of their importance in developing a sound tuberculosis program for the future."[4] To the extent that maximal therapeutic and prophylactic efforts must be directed at people in the ghetto-poverty areas, and must enlist active local participation and support in order to reach both the hard-core resistive active tuberculous and the larger high-risk infected but inactive population, accommodation to community priorities, which do not currently favor personal health services or public health services, will be necessary.

SOME CONCLUDING GENERALIZATIONS

A decade and a half of experience with isoniazid have demonstrated the essential limitations of technological resolutions which, in solving one set of scientific problems, no matter how basic, produce a new set of institutional obstacles to their application and/or reveal deep-rooted social factors that have persistently supported the biological organism and not only fail to yield to a clinical antagonist but actively intervene against its optimal utilization. Additionally, there are difficulties intrinsic to the therapy that minimize its efficacy. Probably the implementation of a single universal one-time intervention is relatively easy to accomplish—such as smallpox vaccination, the immunization of infants against childhood infections, most recently the administration of polio vaccine to all the nation's children. Vigorous and uninterrupted adherence to a long-term course of daily medication, not always without side effects, by apparently healthy individuals who are symptom-free, requires either a high degree of self-discipline and motivation or reliable supervision. The first is not always present in the tuberculosis population, and the second is lacking. We have no manpower resources currently available to work effectively with depressed ghetto patient groups.

Five conclusions in summary:

1. Tuberculosis has traditionally been recognized as a social disease, but little effort has been devoted to developing social solutions. Despite the absence of evidence of causality between disease activation and socioeconomic factors such as poor housing, underemployment, and poverty, the association of tuberculosis with deprivation argues for the need to pursue antipoverty objectives. The marked reduction in the incidence of tuberculosis during the period of socioeconomic improvement of the affected urban population from 1900 to World War II likewise suggests the necessity to mitigate social need among the urban poor. A specific medical solution which is completely effective for the infrequent (today) middle-class patient is insufficient for the poor among whom tuberculosis is concentrated as one of multiple interacting threats. For successful intervention in the current phase of the disease, the organization of tuberculosis control must be responsive to the particular conditions for medical services acceptability among ghetto Negroes and Puerto Ricans, who are difficult populations to reach with the customary assumptions, patterns, and vehicles of public health efforts. Aggressive outreach must replace mere availability among multiproblem groups which do not

utilize health services extensively, and tuberculosis control must be integrated or, at least, coordinated with other services that are essential to the community, namely, welfare, schooling, housing. Of critical importance is the utilization, wherever possible, of nonprofessional workers from within the community to undertake unorthodox ways of providing essential health services to recalcitrant individuals.

2. Structural resistances have also been conspicuous in tuberculosis control. Originally devised to satisfy the requirements of a therapeutic regimen based on long-term isolation of the active patient from the community and highly specialized care, the free-standing clinics, separate inpatient facilities, autonomous record keeping, and laboratory services needed for the new therapy have not been linked together into an intramedical system. Optimal practice requires prompt and fluid movement of the patient through various parts of the system for effective continuous treatment, to say nothing of linkages with nonmedical community services that are necessary adjuncts to specific therapy. At its most egregious, we see the dispersion of tuberculosis control in New York City between the Department of Health and the Department of Hospitals, each facility with its own set of services (medical, nursing, social work) operating under separate local and central administrative authority, the whole network nominally coordinated by a city-wide Tuberculosis Control Director, who can exercise marginal influence but little power. While these facilities have enthusiastically integrated chemotherapy into their medical armamentaria, the structural adaptations implicit in its goals have been minimal.

3. Institutional recalcitrance is not limited to the municipal system. Logic suggests that some voluntary hospitals might have developed tuberculosis services, particularly for ambulatory patients, which would be a useful adjunct to the community and in line with current thought on the desirability of comprehensive delivery and the stated goal of ultimately phasing out specialized acute care facilities. To date, these hospitals provide only 26 beds out of a 1,400 total and serve only 300 of the 12,000 clinic patients. This is their response, after more than ten years of exposure to unequivocal recommendations by successive commissions and study groups, and to

the unchallenged assumption that tuberculosis contagion no longer
constitutes a threat to the general hospital population. It is instructive to compare this negative response with the response of the voluntary sector to simultaneous recommendations that they accept
acutely psychotic patients, hitherto equally inadmissible. Psychiatry,
including inpatient care for those with major psychosis, has become
a major service, stimulated by multiple federal grants for research,
training, and demonstration. With no analogous legislated interest
in tuberculosis, no comparable institutional response occurred. Behind the institutional indifference are two key factors: with the per-
fection of antituberculosis technology, the disease entity no longer
interests the medical school and the teaching hospital; and the association of tuberculosis with the socioeconomically depressed gives it
a low priority in the middle-class-oriented community hospital. The
promise of continued Medicaid support gave impetus to the development of the services in comprehensive neighborhood health facilities; with Medicaid retrenchment, this thrust has been seriously
weakened.

4. Tuberculosis control in New York City today represents in
microcosm the more general problem of medical services for the
poor, principally the slum-concentrated minorities who constitute
the population with the highest risk and simultaneously the population most distant from available preventive and therapeutic services.
This situation has posed an almost insoluble paradox to public health
authorities, whose chief thrust has been technologic refinement and
simplification, and the enhancement of institutional, manpower, and
financial resources, to the point where technology has achieved a
remarkably high level of capability, while the resources lag. The lag,
however, is less threatening in terms of actual availability and volume than in the failure of the target population to exploit existent
resources which are, all things considered, not more deficient than
other municipal services.

To reduce tuberculosis in the ghetto to the residual level which is
indicated by current technology requires the incorporation of that
technology within a system designed to serve the target population—
a concept and an approach which have lagged behind other areas of
health service development. By and large, planning for reform within

the system has been confined to fiscal aspects; what is required, however, is imaginative planning to develop new linkages that will have the dual purpose of introducing the deprived population to existent institutions and services and of actually producing these services in ways acceptable to that population. Where experimental approaches have been designed and utilized, they have reportedly received greater consumer acceptability—the Office of Economic Opportunity centers, such as the Gouverneur Health Services Program and the Martin Luther King, Jr. Neighborhood Health Center, are illustrative. And although these centers have encountered critical difficulties, particularly in the areas of financing and as instruments for the shift of political power to local community groups, one central principle that they have uniformly incorporated, the training and utilization of local paramedical manpower, might profitably be extended to provide the outreach and the long-term monitoring and supervision that are the *sine qua non* of effective tuberculosis control. Where departures from the traditional specialized case-finding and treatment of tuberculosis have been attempted, their yield has been exemplary; the home care and ambulatory services at Jacobi and Van Etten hospitals provide a case in point.

5. The current trend toward a degree of decentralization of health services, especially health planning, has particular import for tuberculosis control. Public health programs are, of necessity, dependent upon community involvement; to the extent that the community is indifferent, preventive programs, particularly as they require any extensive effort, can have only limited impact. With the evolution of community action and self-determination movements, leadership constitutes the most potent force for the adoption and implementation of goals that have thus far lagged for lack of informed interest and support.

But there is a more profound lesson that the persistence of tuberculosis presents, and that is that in the current state of medical science purely technologic approaches to disease and health are anachronistic. The translation of scientific advance into effective service is possible only when due consideration is given to social conditions within which disease and the indices of health flourish, persist, decline. In the absence of a minimum effective health system,

categorical disease approaches, which have traditionally characterized public health efforts and in the last several decades of specialization and subspecialization have extended to clinical medicine as well,
are low-yield operations. If the large underserved population is to be
attached effectively, internal coordination and numerous simplified
entry portals into the health complex are required. In addition,
linkages with the numerous social agencies utilized by the affected
population—employment, welfare, housing—particularly for the purpose of outreach within the neighborhood, must be established if
public health goals are to be realized.

10

LESSONS FROM EXPERIENCE

THIS STUDY of urban health services was undertaken with one primary purpose—to discover, if possible, why most of the recommendations proposed by successive groups of medical and community leaders to alter the structure of the health services industry in New York City with an aim of improving the quantity and quality of care were not followed. Of course, some of the recommendations advanced by committees, commissions, study groups, or consultants were adopted and acted upon, but the sweeping proposals for change aimed at the rationalization of two parallel and largely independent hospital systems—the voluntary and the municipal—were not accepted. Despite repeated advice about the desirability of linking more effectively inpatient and ambulatory services, progress was limited. Despite repeated advice to link the diagnostic and therapeutic services provided by the Department of Health in its various clinics with related programs under the auspices of the Department of Hospitals, little was done. While these departments together with two other major medical agencies, the Office of the Chief Medical Examiner and the Community Mental Health Board, were subsumed in a newly created Health Services Administration in 1967, this organizational superstructure has not resulted in any substantial alteration in the way in which each carries out its respective responsibilities. There had long been liaison between the two departments; there continues to be liaison. But effective integration remains a distant goal.

Recently, medical planners and politicians have begun to urge decentralization of medical services and the active engagement of representatives of the community in planning, administering, and overviewing the operation of health care facilities in their neighborhoods. While it would be presumptuous to forecast what the future will bring, the incontestable fact is that as of the beginning of 1970 progress toward decentralization and productive community involvement has been slow indeed.

For a short time after the passage of Medicare and Medicaid there emerged a euphoric belief that at long last the aged and the poor would have an opportunity to enjoy access to quality medical care on a basis of equality with the more affluent members of the community. For a brief period it appeared that the federal and state governments would put enough money into the medical care system to ensure that those with limited or no private means would no longer have to accept the leftovers from the system. Henceforth, it was hoped, they could obtain treatment from private physicians, be treated in voluntary hospitals, and enjoy all, or most, of the perquisites which are enjoyed by those who can pay for their medical care.

But this vision of a new structure collapsed even before all of the building blocks were in place. At both federal and state levels, the legislators looked at the financial costs of the rapidly growing Medicaid system and beat a hasty retreat. The number of potential eligibles was substantially reduced, as was the scope of benefits.

We can see, then, that successive groups of planners and reformers urged alternative actions to accomplish the following three objectives: to broaden the access of the poor to quality medical services; to improve the quality of the municipal hospital system which produces more than half of both inpatient and outpatient services received by the city's poor; and to rationalize the hydra-headed structure through which health and medical services are provided to the entire community so that the quality of the output can be raised and the costs of operating the system kept within bounds.

It would be difficult to identify any group of informed and interested citizens who would not have given their approval to these three objectives. There was a broad consensus that, while some of the poor were receiving reasonably adequate medical care, a great many had limited access to the system and the quality of care which they received was indifferent and often poor.

While some municipal hospitals were better staffed and run than others, even their ardent supporters never denied that in many the plant was old and undermaintained, the professional leadership weak, the house staff skewed in the direction of poorly trained immigrant physicians, the supporting manpower poorly trained and poorly supervised, essential equipment lacking or out of commission, and that, as a consequence, many patients received an inferior level of care.

With respect to the parallel operation of two largely independent hospital systems, there was broad agreement among informed persons that the pattern resulted in excessive investment of total resources and below-optimum levels of performance. Most observers argued that it was necessary either to obtain better coordination between the two systems or to go the whole way and to integrate them into a single system.

Despite the agreement about the nature of the difficulties and shortcomings in urban health services and about the directions which would have to be followed to reduce and remove the sources of malfunctioning, relatively little progress was made in achieving any of the principal objectives. The poor have remained on the periphery of the system or have been involved in experimental structures designed specifically for them; the municipal hospitals continue to be the subject of apparently justified attack about the quality of services which they render; and the two hospital systems continue to go their independent ways.

Before launching into an analysis of the underlying reasons for this lack of progress we will summarize some of the important changes that have been made in the provision of medical services in New York City during the past decade. We can then expect to see more clearly the conditions that facilitate alterations in the structure in response to pressing needs and opportunities.

The story of what happened and why it happened can be told in terms of three themes: resources, patterns of care, planning. With respect to resources we must pay attention to the following dimensions: manpower, capital, current financing.

Manpower has been enhanced by several major innovations and adaptations made over the past two decades. The establishment of

Albert Einstein College of Medicine and the expansion of Down-state Medical School into one of the largest producers of physicians in the entire country provided two important sources of professional manpower. Through the past associations of Downstate with Kings County Hospital and as a result of careful planning for Einstein and Bronx Municipal Hospital, New York City's municipal hospital system received important reinforcement. Here at least were two hospitals which were not short of good physicians. Whatever other shortcomings there were—and in Kings County the shortcomings were many as a result of overcrowding, decrepit facilities, and other deficiencies—these two hospitals had adequate professional staff in the early 1960s.

Bellevue Hospital is an interesting case in point. After sharing the several services at Bellevue with New York University Medical School for many years, both Columbia and Cornell decided to withdraw. The city had to renegotiate with New York University but it thereby ensured the essential professional staff for the oldest and second largest of its municipal hospitals.

But Kings County, Bronx Municipal, and Bellevue were the exceptions. By the early 1960s, the municipal hospital system confronted a major crisis. Owing, chiefly, to part-time attending staff, the hospitals were unable to attract sufficient interns and residents to provide the basic professional manpower for the several services. The city was faced with operating a hospital system without a medical staff. At this point Commissioner Trussell worked out the first of the affiliation contracts, which provided that each municipal hospital would eventually be linked to a teaching hospital or strong voluntary hospital which would assume the responsibility to provide chiefs of service and house staff, and would ensure control over and general responsibility for the quality of professional services.

There are many questions about how these affiliation contracts worked out over time in terms of cost, the quality of medical care, public control, and other facets of the relationship. But they did provide a partial solution to a major manpower crisis. They offered an interim solution to the problem of keeping the municipal system afloat at a time when it was going under as a consequence of loss of professional manpower. In 1969 the major municipal hospitals were able to attract almost their entire quota of interns under the matching plan, whereas a decade earlier some of them had not attracted a single one!

While the attraction and retention of adequate physician manpower in the municipal hospital system represented the single largest challenge in recent years to the effective operation of health services in New York City, it was by no means the only challenge. There have been chronic shortages of nursing personnel throughout the entire hospital system, voluntary as well as municipal, and shortages, many of them for long periods of time, in allied health manpower—from X-ray technicians to various categories of laboratory personnel.

The crux of these personnel difficulties reflects such diverse factors as the rapid increase in demand for health services; the slow adaptation of wages and salaries in the face of alternative employment opportunities; the growing awareness on the part of hospitals that the operation of a nursing school is likely to result in significant financial loss; persistence of antiquated managerial and guild practices that interfered with optimal utilization of manpower.

Despite these difficulties, it is important to stress how well the "system" adapted so that the required manpower was obtained. The fact that the operation of a nursing school turned from a profitable into an unprofitable undertaking did not lead to closures that would have resulted in large-scale losses of nurses. Several hospitals phased out their programs and a few others that might have started one refrained, but for the most part the existing hospital training structure was maintained and continued to produce approximately the same numbers with a shift toward more nurses who had completed their baccalaureate degrees.

New training structures were put in place and expanded. In particular, the last two decades have seen a substantial expansion of nurse training under vocational education and under the auspices of community and senior colleges. In addition, the new federal manpower training programs, particularly those under the Manpower Development and Training Act, helped to enlarge the health training structure.

Much the same occurred in the case of allied health manpower, although in this instance the hospitals have played the dominant role in the expanded effort. Steps are now under way, however, to broaden and deepen the contribution of the higher educational establishment, notably the City University, to the training of allied health manpower.

No expansion of the training effort alone would have met the expanded demand for medical manpower. In a metropolitan labor market that experienced a strengthened demand in many other sectors, it became essential for the health services industry to establish wages and working conditions that were the approximate equal of what health personnel could secure elsewhere. While the adjustment process was difficult, the fact is that the nursing profession finally did achieve marked gains in salaries and working conditions until nurses now enjoy approximately the position held by other female employees with comparable background and accomplishment. The one claim that the nurses may still advance for further increases relates to the importance and difficulty of their work. But the matter is not as clear as the leadership claims.

With respect to the large and heterogeneous groups subsumed under the heading of "allied health manpower," the trends are less clear. Their salaries increased and their working conditions improved, but these gains probably lagged behind those negotiated by nurses or by the entry-level nontechnical personnel. For a long time the latter were poorly recompensed, but they have made substantial gains in recent years as a consequence of an ever-tighter market for unskilled manpower, trade union organization, and additional third-party money, particularly the flow from the federal government into the hospital system. The latest negotiations, completed in the early fall of 1969 with a group of proprietary hospitals, set a weekly minimum of $125 with additional valuable fringe benefits for housekeeping personnel. It was less than a decade ago that the average wage of this group of hospital employees was in the neighborhood of $50 weekly. Although inflation has eroded part of these gains, the unskilled have secured important advances in real wages.

There is probably no large medical institution in New York City that is fully satisfied with its manpower situation. But the critical question is whether these institutions have unspent personnel funds. The odds are that most do not. The next question is whether, owing to imperfections in the market place, they are forced to pay exorbitant wages or salaries to those whom they hire and consequently cannot cover all their needs. This hardly seems to apply to nurses and allied health manpower, even after taking into consideration the substantial advances which these groups have achieved in recent years. Among physicians, some continue to donate their services; the full-time staff members are paid in relation to what they could earn outside the hospital; and interns' and residents' salaries, while greatly increased over earlier levels, are still below comparable earnings of recent graduates from law schools, engineering schools, and other professional schools.

The simple answer is that through affiliation contracts, the expansion of the training structures, and adjustments in wages and working conditions the health services industry has done remarkably well in securing the requisite manpower (within its budgetary capabilities) to discharge its expanding functions. One further aspect of manpower should be noted. In meeting its manpower requirements the health services industry has taken the lead in attracting large numbers from minority groups by providing reasonably attractive employment opportunities. In this respect it is much further advanced than most sectors of New York industry. It has obtained access to a critically important segment of the potentially available supply, and, furthermore, it has made an important if indirect contribution to helping the disadvantaged populations find a worthwhile place in the economy of New York City.

Capital is the second major aspect of the resource problem. Relatively little money came into New York City from the federal government because the thrust of the Hill-Burton program was directed to areas of low income and low population densities. However, the direct contribution of the federal government to the medical capital plant in New York City goes beyond Hill-Burton monies and includes the significant sums made available for research facilities at the several medical schools and teaching hospitals as well as additional sums under such special programs as community mental health centers. But even when the full gamut of federal funding for capital purposes is taken into consideration the total impact of Washington on the city's health care has been relatively modest.

The same general statement holds for the state government except for its expenditures for the mental hospitals for which it is directly responsible. The state has made selective contributions for hospital construction; it has assisted, through special campus housing programs, the construction of health-related institutions, such as residences for nurses; and recently it has passed special legislation aimed at erecting or rehabilitating hospital and health facilities which will be leased to municipal governments. In New York, the city will eventually be able to acquire the hospitals that the state will build. The value of facilities in various stages of construction under this program approximates $300 million.

For the voluntary sector the primary source of capital funding has continued to be donations from the public through special drives, supplemented by significant gifts from private benefactors and from organized philanthropy. Resort to mortgage loans is a recent development. For the municipal sector, primary responsibility has continued to rest with the government of the City of New York. In both instances the sums that have been raised have not been adequate to provide for new structures to care for burgeoning neighborhoods or for new functions, such as the Mount Sinai School of Medicine, and at the same time to provide adequate sums for maintenance. While the experts differ in their estimates, there is a broad consensus that the hospital plant in New York City, voluntary and municipal, is undermaintained. More serious, much of it is obsolete and should be replaced immediately; other large segments will soon be obsolete unless major renovations and improvements are introduced.

But the required sums are not available, nor are they likely to be forthcoming in the near future. In addition to severe competition for the tax dollar, the costs of construction have risen so steeply that the gap between need and the prospect of meeting it has widened considerably. However, the voluntary sector will be able soon to borrow from the state under favorable terms for construction and rehabilitation.

One favorable development must be noted. In recent years, third-party groups—insurance and government—have been increasingly willing to recognize that depreciation is a proper charge for hospitals to include in their costs for which they seek reimbursement. The conventional figure is 6 percent of allowable costs. Moreover, the hospitals understand that the prospect that third parties will recognize and reimburse this cost is greater if they establish separate depreciation accounts which will be used specifically for rehabilitation.

The present sorry state of the physical plant of the municipal hospital system reflects not only the chronic financial pressures under which New York has long operated but antiquated construction and worse maintenance.

Politicians have also learned to get considerable mileage from the elongated construction process from initial assessment, to letting of contracts, to cornerstone laying, to dedicating the building, to initiating operations. Since a hospital or other type of health facility creates a new financial liability on the operating budget as of the moment that it becomes operational—the city must provide manpower, supplies, and the other essential resources—and since the operating budget is always tight, here is a further reason for slippage.

There is another reason beyond chronic financial stringencies for such slippage. The complex of rules and regulations governing building and supervision; the multiplicity of municipal agencies that have specific responsibilities in the construction of hospitals; and the historic difficulties of obtaining effective coordination among largely independent bureaucracies surely carry much of the onus. The state legislature sought to provide an escape from this dilemma when it acted favorably on the recommendations of the mayor, who had been counseled by the Piel Commission to establish a new agency, the New York City Health and Hospitals Corporation. It remains to be seen whether, in the face of severe financial pressures, the Corporation will in fact be able to perform as effectively as its supporters hope.

The third facet of the resource dimension of medical care relates to the flow of operating funds. This is what we find. Despite the uninhibited escalation of hospital costs, the voluntary part of the system was able to keep increasing its charges to cover steeply mounting per diem costs during the 1950s and 1960s. In turn, Blue Cross and commercial insurance were able to increase their premiums so that they could keep pace with rising hospital reimbursement rates. The city, responding to strong pressure from the voluntary sector, raised its payments for patients for whom it was responsible who were treated outside its own hospitals. Thus the voluntary system was able to make ends meet—although it had to effect economies by delayed maintenance and, for a time, lagging wage and salary levels.

With the introduction of Medicare and Medicaid in 1966, substantial new governmental money was infused into the hospital system, greatly easing the financial burden on voluntary hospitals and the city's budget. Many services that had previously been rendered free or far below cost were now charged at cost and were reimbursed by Medicare or Medicaid. The new monies made it possible for both voluntary and municipal hospitals to meet the demands of nonprofessional workers for substantial raises in their wages, and at the same time they were in a position to increase substantially the pay of interns, residents, and other members of the professional staff for many services for which they had previously donated their time or for which they had earlier received only a modest recompense.

While the financial impact of the new legislation on the municipal system is difficult to isolate because of the flow of funds into and out of different accounts, the following generalizations can be ventured. First, as noted above, the new funds made it possible for the municipal system to raise wages and salaries substantially, thereby slowing, if not stopping, the flow of personnel out of the system. Next, there was some shifting, for a time, of in- and out-patients from municipal hospitals to voluntary institutions and to private practitioners, which reduced the utilization of the municipal system. Finally, when fiscal responsibility for older and medically indigent patients was transferred to the state and federal governments, the city was able to increase expenditures for care of the indigent by more than $40 million while reducing its general tax levy contribution by an almost equal amount.

For a short time it looked as if the ever-present scramble for operating funds for hospital care that confronted both the voluntary system and the city would be permanently eased by the willingness of the state and federal governments to assume such a large part of the total responsibility. But this vision quickly turned into a mirage.

Both Washington and Albany reneged on their initial commitments and the two hospital systems were left in almost as bad shape as earlier. As noted above, the hospitals had quickly adjusted to a higher level of income, and when their new sources of funding were suddenly cut back they were caught in a serious financial squeeze.

One demonstration of the new squeeze for operating funds was the recent request of the New York City Blue Cross for a 43 percent hike in premiums and the ensuing wave of consumer protest which precipitated the issue into the courts. The financial underpinnings of the system of hospital care have been weakened to a point where interest in a comprehensive national system of hospital and health care insurance has been reawakened. While the future will almost certainly bring changes in financing, it is clear that the market mechanisms and governmental actions during the past two decades did provide for the infusion of sufficiently large additional sums to cover the rapidly rising costs and enabled the two hospital systems to remain financially solvent, although the municipal system was not able to bring its quality of care to an acceptable level.

While manpower, facilities, and money are the critical resources required for the provision of health and hospital services, the ways in which they are used and managed have much to do with the outcome. Hence we must now attend briefly to the changes which took place in the patterns of medical care. In this connection we will review what happened on three fronts: emergency room care, ambulatory care, and the adaptations in the treatment of patients with tuberculosis following the chemotherapeutic breakthrough of the early 1950s.

There are two ways of reading the story of the expansion of emergency room care. Some observers believe that it represented little that was new. Hospitals had always treated patients who walked in off the street. The last decades, say this group, have seen an expansion of this long-established pattern. The fact that many hospitals, despite a growing work load, have made relatively few adjustments in facilities, staffing, management, and financing of emergency room services reinforces the claims of those who see nothing significant in this development.

But there is a second view, for which we opt. The scale of the expansion in emergency room care is proof that a new and important change has in fact occurred. Many consumers, especially those in low-income brackets, balked by their inability to find a physician when they needed one, increasingly brought their medical problems to the hospital. Since most hospitals, for professional and public relations reasons, are loath to turn a patient away because they may be jeopardizing his life if they do, they provide more and more care in the emergency room. Some understood earlier than others that this expansion was an important new dimension of their work and instituted appropriate changes to cope with it. Others came to this realization more slowly. But irrespective of the promptness of the individual hospital's response, the unequivocal fact is that the rapid expansion of emergency room services is a case illustration of how the uncoordinated actions of hard-pressed consumers forced a significant alteration in the pattern of medical care. The two other factors that contributed to this innovation were the willingness of many physicians to encourage the pattern and the relative ease with which many hospitals absorbed the additional load by adapting facilities and instituting staffing changes.

For many years the large teaching hospital in an urban community has provided ambulatory services to the poor both as a contribution to neighborhood medicine and as a necessary adjunct to its teaching program. The outpatient clinic served as a screening and evaluating mechanism to determine which patients should be admitted to the wards for further treatment where they would provide the clinical material for teaching purposes.

But this pattern, whereby the teaching hospital provided both ambulatory and inpatient care to the poor, has not been generalized to include the bulk of the patient population who pay their own way and who select their own physician. While medical planners have stressed the gains that could accrue from rationalizing inpatient and outpatient care, gains by both professional and financial criteria, progress has been slow.

The reasons are not hard to uncover. Conventional insurance policies—though not major medical, HIP, or GHI—cover inpatient care only. Hence both patient and physician have a bias in that direction. Large urban hospitals, while they may have a few full-time staff members, make their facilities available to large numbers of physicians in the community who have been granted staff privileges. There is no easy way, in fact there is no way, for such a hospital to expand its ambulatory services without running headlong into conflict with the community physician. Either he treats his patient or the hospital's full-time staff does. And he who performs the treatment gets the fee!

Medical idealists have argued for years that better integration of in- and outpatient care requires that the potential patient be a member of a comprehensive prepaid insurance plan. Then, and only then, will sound decisions be made as to the locus of treatment—in the physician's office, the hospital's outpatient department, its inpatient facilities, or at a medical center. But this preferred approach requires not only prepaid group practice but preferably a hospital controlled by the group, for otherwise there will be conflict over the division of the dollar.

The story in New York City is as follows. Two principal prepaid insurance systems have been in operation—HIP and GHI—throughout the last two decades. While each has grown, the rate of growth in the most recent period has been minimal. Many of the groups in the HIP system have had difficulties in attracting and retaining competent physicians at the salaries that they have been able to pay. HIP has also been handicapped in developing effective hospital linkages. While HIP recently acquired LaGuardia Hospital in Queens, the plan's only prior hospital linkage (Montefiore) has just been cut because the hospital contended that HIP's reimbursement rates were so low that they created a severe operating deficit.

Without delving deeper into the constraints on the growth of HIP in the New York City area, suffice it to say in the present context that the last two decades have seen remarkably little innovation in the provision of ambulatory services for the paying patient. The changes which were introduced were limited almost exclusively to experiments directed at helping the poor.

Recently various insurance systems, other than major medical, have begun, gingerly, to experiment with new policies that will provide a limited amount of ambulatory services. These underwriters recognize the potential advantages to claimant and insurer if it proves possible to deter patients from seeking hospitalization for diagnostic or therapeutic procedures that could be provided efficiently on an outpatient basis. But the insurance companies are moving slowly because of the need to differentiate between open-ended physician care and specifically delineated ambulatory services provided at a hospital. The line between these two will not be easy to draw. The probability is strong, therefore, that while much will still be written about the desirability of closer integration between in- and outpatient services, additional experimentation will involve primarily the poor, whose financial conditions, at least in terms of physicians' earnings, are unimportant or nonexistent.

The early 1950s saw one of the spectacular breakthroughs in modern medicine. Although tuberculosis was not the scourge that it had been earlier in the century, it continued to afflict large numbers of people. And until the introduction of isoniazid, the preferred therapy had been hospital and sanatorium bed rest. With the breakthrough, the tuberculosis patient required only a brief period of bed rest while his active infection was brought under control; thereafter he could complete his therapy on an ambulatory basis.

So dramatic a change in the treatment of a disease required a great number of adjustments in the operations of hospitals, clinics, and professional and supporting staffs. While many of these adjustments were made, such as, for instance, the striking decline in tuberculosis bed capacity in the municipal hospitals, many others were not introduced or were introduced slowly. The voluntary hospitals would not treat tuberculosis patients. The Health Department's tuberculosis clinics and the Hospital Department's in- and outpatient efforts were not effectively correlated. Many hospital directors were skittish about speeding the release of patients, fearful that they would be lost to therapy upon release. Only one hospital undertook a comprehensive demonstration program, including social work with the family, to test the limits of early hospital release. Despite the predominance of minority groups among the tuberculosis patient population, the medical authorities shied away from involving these groups in preventive and therapeutic programming.

In 1970 the treatment of tuberculosis is much improved over 1950 before the new drugs made their appearance. But a critical review of the present pattern of diagnosis and treatment underscores the fact that the dead hand of the past continues strong because of the absence of any effective leverage to speed desirable changes in hospital, clinic, and community programming. Among the principal reasons for the slow rate of change are the absence of additional funds to exploit fully the potentialities of the new approaches; the inherent difficulties of modifying the ideas and practices of a deeply entrenched bureaucracy; and the lack of imagination among the professional leadership about the desirability of involving the community.

To the extent that changes in emergency room services, ambulatory care, and the care of patients with tuberculosis provide a testing of the alternatives in the pattern of medical care in the last two decades the following conclusions are suggested. It is easier to innovate in the treatment of patients who generally do not pay for their care, for example, the bulk of emergency room cases, than it is when the conventional financial relations between patient and physician are likely to be affected, as in the case of private ambulatory patients. Even when a scientific breakthrough occurs, as in the treatment of tuberculosis, it is difficult to exploit it quickly and effectively because of the shortages of funds and the resistance on the part of the medical establishment to restructure the therapeutic regimen and to make use of nonprofessionals, particularly indigenous workers, in unconventional ways. Finally, changes in the patterning of care are not likely to be introduced on the grounds of economy or efficiency if the prevailing system demonstrates reasonable viability, which in fact it did during this period.

We now confront the third and last dimension of the study of change—an evaluation of the planning function. First, a few words about the planning organizations which were in place at the end of World War II or shortly thereafter. The most important agency was the Health and Hospital Planning Council of Southern New York, the metropolitan hospital planning council that came into being in the late 1930s and that acquired quasi-governmental responsibilities after World War II when it was authorized by the state of New York to approve projects seeking Hill-Burton support. In the late 1960s it was given additional powers under expanded state-regulating authority; no additional bed capacity could be added by a hospital unless it had the prior approval of the Hospital Council.

While the Council was dominated by the voluntary sector, it did include as members of its board of directors the principal health and hospital officials of New York City. However, when the federal government under recent legislation (Public Law 89-749) made new funds available for comprehensive health planning subject to the establishment of a single planning agency, a protracted struggle developed between the City of New York and the Council for designation by the state. The first round was won by the city, which is proceeding with the organization of a comprehensive planning unit for the region.

The intensity of the struggle and the inability of the two contesting parties to compromise their differences reflect the deep mutual suspicion between voluntary sector and government—suspicion that grew out of the past relations of the Council and government. The city believes that the Council has always done the bidding of the voluntary sector. In doing so it has failed to take effective leadership in rationalizing the two hospital systems. For the most part it has taken only those actions aimed at strengthening the independence of the private sector. On the other hand, the voluntary sector, seeing the increasingly serious plight into which the hospital services and lately even the health services of the city have fallen, has been concerned that municipal leadership of the hospital system might result in a mandatory sharing of the wealth, which would require an outflow of financial and manpower resources from the voluntary sector to shore up the poorly functioning city hospital system. Hence the voluntary institutions have been determined to avoid a closer relationship with the city than the narrowly defined affiliations whereby they provide professional staff or hospital care under carefully stipulated contractual arrangements.

With this condensed summary of action and reaction between the two sectors—voluntary and governmental—we can conclude that over the last two decades political power was so distributed that the voluntary hospitals were able to avoid encroachment on their historic preserves by the Council through its planning function. One or another voluntary hospital made requests of a technical nature of the Council from time to time. And the Council periodically undertook studies that involved all hospitals in the region, or a specific geographic or functional subset. But the Council never took action that dealt with the heart of any matter unless the predominant voluntary agencies were in agreement.

Under federal legislation passed in the middle 1960s which supported the development of strong research training and service programs centered on heart disease, cancer, and stroke, the region faced another planning challenge. Once again, it failed. These programs were developed on a medical-school-centered regional model, but in New York City there was not one but six medical schools—Columbia, Cornell, New York University, Albert Einstein, Downstate, New York Medical College—and most recently a seventh—Mount Sinai—with no one dominant. It would probably be an exaggeration to say that nothing was produced by these programs under which approximately $2 million was allocated to the New York area, but it is correct to state that a gap remains between intent and accomplishment. While particular difficulties arise when planning involves both the voluntary and the municipal sector, each with a guarded attitude toward the other, apparently the situation is not much eased when the planning is entrusted to the voluntary sector, which can proceed under its own steam if it is able to agree on objectives and implementation.

A third facet of planning characteristic of the 1960s and once again involving federal financing is represented by the Office of Economic Opportunity grants for the development of neighborhood health centers in low-income areas. The outstanding case is the Martin Luther King, Jr. Neighborhood Health Center linked with Montefiore Hospital. The objective of this new program was to expand and improve ongoing health services for the poor and in the process to engage representatives of the poor in the planning and provision of such services. In both conception and execution the new program was highly innovative. While there had been many earlier attempts to improve health services for the poor, it was a chance to offer them a voice in the direction of the program and an opportunity to be employed on an expanded health team.

The initial planning from Washington looked forward to a series of federally subsidized centers in the New York City area but hardly had the first come into existence than the federal government reconsidered. From the limited experience to date we can say that totally federally subsidized health delivery effort aimed exclusively at the poor has a reasonable chance of support and success—at least in eliciting cooperation from a part of the local medical establishment and from the poor themselves. This is not to say that we know how to balance professional with community leadership; or where to draw the line between specifically health services and socially or politically related supplementary services; or the preferred arrangements for balancing the need of local people for employment and their capability to be productive members of the health team; or how to relate more effectively the new health center to its supporting hospital and to home care programs.

We must also know more about the potential costs and benefits of such new neighborhood centers versus alternative uses of equivalent and—even more important—sustainable sources of governmental revenue aimed at raising the level of health care for the poor. For $1,000 per family per year, there must be more than improved clinic care. The early retreat of the federal government is certainly connected to this critical issue of costs.

The innovative potential of neighborhood centers should not be lost. The demonstrated possibility of improved care for the poor through utilization of the indigenous population as a manpower resource, new tables of organization for health facilities, and new linkages between patient and the system provides options for expanding and reforming the delivery of ambulatory care. These innovations should be considered and acted upon as a means of increasing access and effectiveness if the costs can be held within reasonable bounds.

Finally we must confront an even more basic problem in planning: whether it is sensible and sound to fashion a system of health care for the poor that is substantially independent of the system of care utilized by other members of the community; or whether the poor are likely to do better over time if they can be locked into the same system, with modifications, as that used by the consumer who is able to pay for his care. There is little in the more recent OEO experience that gives much support to the principle of an independent system—once account is taken of the high costs—even while it remains true that many shortcomings and defects continue to exist when the poor must seek care from systems that are geared primarily to provide services for the nonpoor.

There remains one further aspect of health services planning to which the recent New York City experience is apposite: that of regionalization in the borough of the Bronx. In recent years we have seen that when there are points of interest among a dominant group within the voluntary community, such as those represented by the voluntary hospitals associated with the Federation of Jewish Philanthropies; when the same group has control over the local medical school, as with Albert Einstein College of Medicine; when the City of New York has found it desirable to negotiate affiliation contracts (for example, between Montefiore and Morrisania, and between Misericordia and Fordham); when one of the medical institutions has aggressive leadership (for example, Montefiore) and is interested in community experimentation; and when the low-income groups in the neighborhood (that is, Negroes and Puerto Ricans) are in an early stage of political organization—the preconditions exist for bringing about a series of changes aimed at rationalizing via regionalization the provision of medical services throughout the borough. But it is necessary only to set out the complex conditions that must be present in order for such an effort to be ventured and to succeed even partially. Small wonder that regionalization has been much more talked and written about than acted on.

We have sought in this penultimate chapter to recapitulate at a higher level of abstraction what happened—and what failed to happen—in New York City in the last decade or so to alter the pattern of providing and distributing health services to the community. We have seen that it has proved difficult indeed to alter the resources, the patterns of care, and the planning which provide the basic parameters of the system. While changes have occurred in response to emergencies, opportunities, and alternatives in the market place, the outstanding finding is the inertia of the system as a whole.

CONCLUSION: GUIDELINES
FOR PLANNERS

AN EVALUATIVE REVIEW of efforts to improve health services in New York City and of the successes achieved and the failures registered is one important way of acquiring knowledge about the factors which facilitate or retard improvement. In this concluding chapter we will seek to highlight the lessons that were learned so that they can serve as guidelines for planners who will be responsible for the system in the years ahead.

All the evidence supporting the guidelines presented below has been set out and evaluated in earlier chapters; it will therefore be possible to present the following conclusions tersely.

1. *Pluralism operates as both potential for and constraint on reforming the health system.* It is not true, as many believe, that because health services are provided by so many discrete interest groups, including private practitioners, medical schools, government, nonprofit and commercial insurance plans, trade unions, voluntary hospitals, and health organizations, significant reforms cannot be accomplished without comprehensive planning and a comprehensive system for delivering services.

The existence of multiple power centers creates a great many interfaces and frontiers where sovereignty has not yet been claimed. There are therefore important margins where changes can be introduced. And the record over the last two decades reveals many such changes, from the training of allied health manpower to the expansion of emergency room care.

The potentials for constructive reform under pluralism go further. The recent past disclosed that, even in the arenas where powerful groups have entrenched interests, emergencies or new opportunities do arise from time to time which facilitate changes in the structure whereby medical services are produced and distributed, as in the regionalization of the Bronx.

Although pluralism does not prevent change, it points up the difficulties attendant on bringing about large-scale alteration of the status quo. Each of the major parties insists that its essential power remain undiminished as a result of any contemplated large-scale change. While it might be possible to design on paper significant reforms that would protect the interests of all of the major groups, even that would be difficult. Moreover, the expenditures of time and effort required to negotiate changes which meet these conditions must be considered in striking a trial balance between the old and the new. Inherent in pluralism is an overwhelming presumption in favor of incremental rather than large-scale reforms.

2. *The effective power of government to reform the health system is limited.* Despite a substantial drift after World War II in the direction of expanding government's role in the health industry, the simple fact is that the industry remains dominated by the private sector—consumers, private practitioners, voluntary hospitals. Thus, in both legislative and administrative matters, government's scope for changing the system is constrained by the necessity to elicit support from those who will be affected by the changes. While government can find selected issues on which it can gain broad-scale public support and lean successfully against one or another interest group, it will seldom be able to corral the support required to engage several of the groups simultaneously which is the *sine qua non* for instituting broad-scale changes in the system. At least this appears to be the only reasonable deduction as long as the majority of the public is willing to go along with the health care system as it currently operates. In the absence of wide-scale public discontent with the status quo, government has no directive to enter upon designing and implementing radical new programs.

3. *The effectiveness of government's intervention depends on its strategy and tactics.* Since most good hospital care is provided by nonprofit hospitals, the parallel operation of hospitals under governmental aegis is likely to result in wasteful use of resources, selective

admission policies, or different levels of patient care—or all three. Government should avoid expanding its operational responsibilities for providing hospital care and seek to reduce its direct operational involvement. In the interim it should aim to make its hospitals part of a coordinated system by subspecialization and closer linkages with the voluntary sector. Government can usually reduce its expenditures for hospital care by buying services for specified groups in the population for whom it has responsibility. State government might insist upon compulsory hospital insurance, possibly with selective subsidization, to reduce to a minimum the number of potential welfare cases for whose hospitalization it must pay. Tax credits for hospital and health insurance should be avoided because of the dangers inherent in further erosion of the tax base, because such credits will fail to ensure maximum enrollments of the potentially coverable population, and because they will provide a subsidy to higher-income groups.

4. *Improvements in the health system require improvements in planning and evaluation.* One of the untoward results of pluralism has been the slow growth of planning and evaluation mechanisms. Each of the principal groups has sought to maintain maximum autonomy. The more productive use of resources requires that future investments be made with an eye to the requirements of the community as a whole and that evaluation mechanisms be established to assess the results of these investments. Since decision-making for the expansion and operation of the health system is splintered, the planning agency must include representatives from the principally concerned sectors, but to be effective the agency must have governmental and public support to enforce its decisions. With respect to evaluation, the public that uses the services, third parties that foot much of the bill, and the leaders of the several professions involved who are in the best position to assess the quality of the outcomes must all play a part. Regular reporting to the community is an essential aspect of both improved planning and evaluation.

5. *Basic and applied research capabilities in health systems analysis must be strengthened.* The scale and complexity of modern systems of providing health services point up the urgent necessity to broaden and deepen research so that decision-making can be

strengthened. Hospitals represent large sunk costs. Hence decisions about where to build, what to build, and the range of services to be provided should be made in light of the best estimates of present needs and prospective changes in the community. Power when faced with facts is likely to be less arbitrary than when it operates in the dark. Moreover, constant changes in medical knowledge and technology point to the desirability that researchers explore how the system can be adapted to such changes. Similarly, constant changes in demographic, social, and economic conditions need to be monitored so that the health service structure can be responsive. While each of the powerful interest groups, as well as planning and evaluation agencies, needs an in-house research capability, a substantial broadening of the total research effort is required. To fulfill its potential such an effort should be carried out under university or other independent auspices, but it might be supported in part by the principal interested groups.

6. *Experimental and demonstration projects should be initiated only after long-term financing prospects have been explored and provision made for evaluation.* The last several years have seen the launching of a considerable number of experimental and demonstration projects aimed at improving the delivery of medical services, particularly to the poor. In many instances little constraint existed on the cost of providing these improved services since the projects were experimental. This situation should be avoided in the future because such experiments raise false expectations. If they are successful it is anticipated that they will be continued, which often is not possible, or that they will be replicated elsewhere, which also is not possible because of lack of funding. If government is the sponsor, the pressure to continue a successful experiment that has gained broad visibility is great indeed. Often government is forced to keep the project alive even though a redirection of resources would yield much higher benefits.

7. *Preference should be given to modifying existing institutions rather than adding new ones to the health system.* It is generally easier in both the public and the private sector to add a new institution to meet new or expanding needs than to bring about changes in the existing institutions. Because of the long-term commitments to,

and the interests of staff in, particular clienteles, doctors, and methods of operations, a high order of leadership is required to attempt to change a part of the establishment that has a record of service and accomplishment. But unless modifications in existing institutions are ventured and succeed, the costs of operating the medical care system will mount steeply and the productivity of the system will be far below optimum because of the constant accretion of new institutions to meet new needs. One of the consequences of medical and social progress is the elimination over time of needs that were once primary. To leave the existing structure more or less intact is to ensure that it will be operated at lower effectiveness.

8. *There is need to establish closer relations between budgeting for capital and operating purposes.* Because of the critical part that hospitals and related health institutions have played and continue to play in the provision of health services, the attention of politicians, planners, and the public has been riveted on securing the required capital for constructing new institutions and outfitting them. This preoccupation with capital requirements has frequently obscured the fact that, without adequate sources of finances and manpower to operate the institution effectively, the structure will be unable to contribute significantly to meeting the community's needs. Government in particular tends to focus unduly on capital to the neglect of operating needs, neglecting the fact that the costs of operating a hospital bed for a little more than one year equal or exceed its capital cost. In a fully employed, even overemployed, medical manpower economy there is a further danger that even if operating funds are available when a new institution comes on stream it may prove difficult to recruit the required numbers of qualified personnel. Effective budgeting means that the requirements for capital, operating funds, and manpower must be considered as an entity. The quantity and quality of the services may be more effectively increased by avoiding new construction in favor of alternative investments to modernize existing plant or strengthen existing staff resources.

9. *It is wrong for planners and politicians to promise a single standard of high-level medical care for all citizens.* In a society in which there are gross discrepancies in the quantity and quality of health services being provided to different communities and to dif-

ferent groups within the same community in which there are scarcities of medical manpower and in which there is intensive competition for the tax dollar, there is no prospect of fulfilling a promise of a single standard of high-quality medical care for all. Moreover, this could not be guaranteed even if government were to give the highest priority to funding health services. The unequal distribution of income would still result in wealthy people being able to command more of the limited pool of quality medical resources. Only a radical new system involving compulsion with respect to the attraction of professional manpower and the ability to control patient assignments could move significantly toward realizing such an objective. In the absence of radical reforms, it is preferable to formulate goals more in consonance with the potentiality of realizing them, such as aiming to ensure that the poor will have access to essential health services.

10. *A bifurcated health system, one for the middle and upper classes and the other for the poor, is inefficient.* While it may not be possible for society to provide a single system of superior health services for all in the foreseeable future, it is important to recognize that separate systems for middle class and poor are inequitable and inefficient. It has not been possible in the past and there is no ground for believing that it will be possible in the future for the system which cares for the poor to attract the financial and particularly the manpower resources that are required to provide the poor with the range of services that they require. The best prospect for improving the quality of services available to the poor is to lock them into the same system that cares for the middle class and to make adaptations in that system so that it will be better able to cope with their special needs. This means that it is generally preferable to expand the access of the poor to ambulatory and inpatient services of well-run hospitals, adding special staffs of indigenous workers to facilitate improved communication and utilization, than to construct a special group of medical institutions to serve the poor exclusively.

11. *In the provision of health services there is a danger that the input of additional resources will be equated with the output of additional services.* The last years have seen the investment of considerably larger amounts of governmental funds in the health system on

the presumption that these will be reflected in the provision of additional services. Even though government made it possible for the poor to pay for health services, it does not follow that all or even most of the poor succeeded in gaining access to improved services. One important reason is that many of the purveyors of service—hospitals, clinics, physicians, and others—raised their charges and fees. Given the imperfections of the health market, it behooves government to make additional financial resources available only as it can use them to bargain for changes in the institutional structures aimed at an enlarged output and a better distribution of services.

12. *The health system is not self-contained; its ability to provide more and better services depends on improved linkages with other systems.* When a sector of society finds that it is handicapped in accomplishing its goals, it tends to reach out and aims to do more. While the effective rehabilitation of a tuberculosis patient may require social work services, such as finding a new apartment or getting the patient a suitable job, it does not follow that a hospital and health system must extend its boundaries until it has its own social welfare, housing, and employment units. The key challenge that it faces here is to improve its linkages with other systems that can contribute to the desired ends. The relative isolation that has characterized medicine in the past suggests that significant gains lie ahead if proper linkages can be established with such important systems as education and manpower training, employment, social welfare, and transportation.

13. *There is need for an improved method for selecting targets for reform.* Since there are wide gaps between the goals of a quality health system and the performance of the existing one, there is a crowded agenda of changes that might be introduced. But the critical challenge that faces different communities and the nation at large is to make a selection among the alternative targets. One criterion is the potential gains that will follow upon the introduction of specific improvements. But it is essential that another criterion be applied: the probability, in a pluralistic system, of succeeding in making a particular change. If the probability is low, then it may be advisable to select an area where the particular gains may be less but are more certain.

14. *A system of national health insurance, even if passed in the next few years, will not ensure that the urban population will secure access to quality health services.* The present bills in Congress contemplate a reallocation of present expenditures, no increase in the levels of spending. They assume that the rapid expansion of comprehensive prepaid health programs will result in marked economies and efficiencies sufficient to provide the additional resources required for expanding services to the poor and the self-supporting. There is no likelihood that such radical changes in the output of health services can be accomplished solely by relying on the pressures and incentives contained in the pending legislation. Moreover, the absence of available infrastructure—comprehensive clinics, community hospitals, other basic facilities and staff—precludes the likelihood of realizing such an ambitious goal. There is good reason to suggest that alternative measures of reform, specifically directed to high-priority objectives such as expanding access for the poor into the mainstream of medicine for basic care, would have more prospect of accomplishment and avoid the dangers of counterproductive changes.

15. *Political leadership and administrative stability are important ingredients in accomplishing significant improvements in the health system.* There is little point for any group, governmental or private, to seek to launch a program of health reform unless it can gain the wholehearted support of its leadership. It is difficult in a pluralistic system to convince the key interest groups to alter their goals or methods of operation. Hence a strong commitment of the leadership is the *sine qua non* of success. An important secondary factor is a friendly or at least nonhostile bureaucracy. Because of the time dimensions required to carry out a significant reform program in the health field from conception to implementation, a sympathetic bureaucracy is essential.

NOTES AND REFERENCES

CHAPTER 2. EXPANDING MANPOWER RESOURCES

1. Board of Higher Education, *Master Plan of the Board of Higher Education for the City University of New York, 1968* (New York: Board of Higher Education, 1968), p. 225.
2. Harold Rowe, "Estimates of Costs of Nursing Programs," in Hospital Review and Planning Council of Southern New York, *Study of Nurse Education Needs in Southern New York Region* (New York: Hospital Review and Planning Council, April, 1967) pp. 128-31.
3. Office of the Dean for Community College Affairs of the CUNY, *A Proposal for the Establishment of Community College Number Eight* (New York: Board of Higher Education, April, 1968).
4. "City U. Planning Harlem Branch," New York *Times,* July 6, 1968, p. 1.
5. Department of Hospitals of the City of New York and District Council No. 37, "An Upgrading Promotion and Training Program for Nurse's Aides" (New York: District Council No. 37, n.d.); Sumner Rosen, "Building Career Ladders in Health Occupations—Opportunities and Obstacles" (New York: New Careers Development Center, n.d.); Richard Bumstead, "LPN Training: It's Worth the Struggle," *Training,* April, 1968.
6. Eleanor Gilpatrick, *Train Practical Nurses to Become Registered Nurses: A Survey of the PN Point of View* (Health Services Mobility Study, Research Report No. 1 [New York: Research Foundation, City University of New York, June, 1968]).
7. Albert Einstein College of Medicine–Lincoln Hospital Health Careers Program, *Transitional Report,* April 1, 1968.
8. Eleanor Gilpatrick and Paul Corliss, *The Occupational Structure of New York City Municipal Hospitals* (Health Services Mobility Study, Research Report No. 2 [New York: Research Foundation, City University of New York, 1969]), p. 33.
9. This discussion is based on information supplied by the Bureau of X-Ray Technology, New York State Department of Health.

10. The annual issues of the National League for Nursing, *State Approved Schools of Nursing—LPN.*

11. Based on material prepared by the New York State Optometric Association and a discussion with Dr. Alden Haffner, Director, Optometric Center of New York.

12. American Nurses' Association, *Facts About Nursing: A Statistical Summary,* 1968 edition, (New York: American Nurses' Association), pp. 53-60.

CHAPTER 3. CAPITAL FUNDING

1. *Appraisal of Hospital Obsolescence,* Special Report No. 4, Hospital Review and Planning Council of Southern New York, Inc., 1965.

2. Herbert E. Klarman, *Hospital Care in New York City* (New York: Columbia University Press, 1963), Table 8-16, p. 270.

3. New York *Times,* October 8, 1969, and Dr. Mary McLaughlin, "Current Status and Problems of New York City's Comprehensive Neighborhood Family Care Health Centers," presented at the Annual Health Conference of the New York Academy of Medicine, April 26, 1968.

4. Klarman, *Hospital Care,* p. 256.

5. C. Rufus Rorem, *Capital Financing for Hospitals* (New York: Health and Hospital Planning Council of Southern New York, Inc., June, 1968), Table VI, p. 16.

6. *Appraisal of Hospital Obsolescence,* p. 41.

7. Rorem, *Capital Financing for Hospitals,* p. 15.

8. Paul Worthington, personal communication, May 27, 1969.

9. Charlotte Muller and Paul Worthington, "Factors Entering into Capital Decisions of Hospitals," paper prepared for the Second Conference on the Economics of Health at the Johns Hopkins University, December, 1968.

CHAPTER 6. EMERGENCY ROOM SERVICES

1. E. R. Weinerman, R. S. Ratner, A. Robbins, and M. A. Lavenhar, "Yale Studies in Ambulatory Medical Care. V. Determinants of Use of Hospital Emergency Services," *American Journal of Public Health,* LVI (July, 1966), 1037; AMA Dept. of Hospital and Medical Facilities, "The Emergency Department Problem," *Journal of the American Medical Association,* October 24, 1966; J. Reed and G. Reader, "Quantitative Survey of New York Hospital Emergency Room, 1965," *New York State Journal of Medicine,* May 15, 1967.

2. *Accidental Death and Disability: The Neglected Disease of Modern*

Society, monograph by National Academy of Science and National Research Council, Washington, D.C., 1966, p. 8.

3. Paul Torrens, "The Impact of Emergency Services Upon Patterns of Ambulatory Care," report submitted to Medical Care Administrative Branch of Division of Community Health Services, Public Health Service, August, 1965.

4. *Ibid.*

5. Reed and Reader, "Quantitative Survey of New York Hospital Emergency Room, 1965."

6. Haydee Inclan, "Physicians and Dentists in Private Practice in the Gouverneur Medical Service Area, New York City, 1966–1967," Urban Medical Economics Research Project, Urban Research Center, Hunter College, CUNY, 1967.

7. Based upon aggregated data from monthly records kept by the Department of Social Services.

8. United Hospital Fund of New York, "Analysis of Hospital Personnel, 1961–1967."

9. Torrens, "The Impact of Emergency Services upon Patterns of Ambulatory Care."

CHAPTER 8. THE PROCESS OF REGIONALIZATION: THE BRONX

1. Commission on the Delivery of Personal Health Services, *Comprehensive Community Health Services for New York City,* December, 1967, p. 26.

2. In the course of preparing this chapter interviews were held with Dr. Vincent Larkin, former Director of the New York Regional Medical Program; Dr. Shirley Fisk, Regional Medical Program Coordinator for Columbia University; and William Glazier, Regional Medical Program Coordinator for the Albert Einstein College of Medicine.

3. Department of Health, Education, and Welfare, *Obligations to Medical Schools, Fiscal Year 1967* (Washington, D.C.: National Institutes of Health, 1968), p. 4.

4. Eli Ginzberg and Peter Rogatz, *Planning for Better Hospital Care* (New York: Kings Crown Press, 1961).

5. Raymond Lerner, Corinne Kirchner, and Emil Dieckmann, *New York City Municipal General Hospital Outpatient Study, 1965: Data on Social Background, Medical Care Utilization, and Attitude of Outpatients, by Hospital* (New York: School of Public Health and Administrative Medicine of Columbia University, Report No. 3, August, 1968), p. 2.

6. A highly critical paper is Peter Rothstein, "The Closing of St. Francis

Hospital: A Case Study of the Politics of Health Planning" (New York: Health Policy Advisory Center, 1968).

7. Hospital Council of Greater New York, "Report on the Municipal Hospitals in the Bronx" (an unpublished report dated May, 1959).

8. *Milbank Memorial Fund Quarterly*, Vol. XLVI, No. 3 (July, 1968), Part I, is devoted to a discussion of this project. Additional information was obtained during a visit to the center.

9. A schedule of hospital rates is issued periodically by the Office of Health Economics of the New York State Health Department.

CHAPTER 9. TB CONTROL

1. Herbert E. Klarman, *Hospital Care in New York City* (New York: Columbia University Press, 1963), pp. 72-76.

2. Eli Ginzberg, *A Pattern for Hospital Care* (New York: Columbia University Press, 1949), p. 208.

3. Task Force on Tuberculosis in New York City, *A Modern Attack on an Urban Health Problem,* report (December, 1968), p. 25.

4. *Ibid.,* p. 11.

SELECTED BIBLIOGRAPHY

Baumgartner, Leona. "One Hundred Years of Health, New York City 1866 to 1966," *Bulletin of the New York Academy of Medicine*, June, 1969.

Blue Ribbon Panel on Municipal Hospitals of New York City. *Report to Governor Nelson A. Rockefeller.* April, 1967.

Blumenkrantz, Joseph. "Planning Medical Care Facilities: Present Trends and Future Possibilities," *American Journal of Public Health*, Vol. LVI, No. 10 (October, 1966).

Board of Higher Education, City of New York. *Master Plan of the Board of Higher Education for the City University of New York.* New York: Board of Higher Education, 1968.

Burlage, Robb. *New York City's Municipal Hospitals: A Policy Review.* Washington, D.C.: Institute for Policy Studies, May, 1967.

City of New York. *Capital Budget.* Annual, 1960-.

—— *Expense Budget.* Annual, 1960-.

—— Department of Health. *Annual Report.* 1960-.

—— Department of Hospitals. *Annual Report.* 1960-.

—— Office of the Comptroller. *Annual Report.* 1960-.

Commission on Health Services of the City of New York. *Report* (Heyman Report). July 20, 1960.

Commission on the Delivery of Personal Health Services (Piel Commission). *Comprehensive Community Health Services for New York City.* December, 1967.

Division of Research and Statistics, Health Insurance Plan of Greater New York. *Statistical Report.* Annual, 1960-. New York: Health Insurance Plan of Greater New York.

Donabedian, Avedis. "An Evaluation of Prepaid Group Practice," *Inquiry*, September, 1969.

Gilpatrick, Eleanor, and Paul Corliss. *The Occupational Structure of New York City Municipal Hospitals.* Health Services Mobility Study, Research Report No. 2. New York: Research Foundation, City University of New York, 1969.

Ginzberg, Eli. *Men, Money, and Medicine.* New York: Columbia University Press, 1969.

—— A Pattern for Hospital Care. New York: Columbia University Press, 1949.

Ginzberg, Eli, and Peter Rogatz. Planning for Better Hospital Care. New York: Kings Crown Press, 1961.

Goodrich, Charles, Margaret Olendzki, and George Reader. Welfare Medical Care: An Experiment. Cambridge, Mass.: Harvard University Press, 1970.

Governor's Committee on Hospital Costs. Report. December 15, 1965.

Greenfield, Harry, and Carol Brown. Allied Health Manpower: Trends and Prospects. New York: Columbia University Press, 1969.

Health and Hospital Planning Council of Southern New York, Inc. (formerly Hospital Council of Greater New York, 1938 to 1962; Hospital Review and Planning Council of Southern New York, Inc., 1962 to 1967). Annual Report. 1950-.

—— Appraisal of Hospital Obsolescence. 1965.

—— The Hill-Burton Program in Southern New York, 1948-1963. 1964.

—— Hospital Staff Appointments of Physicians in New York City. New York: Macmillan, 1951.

—— Hospitals and Related Facilities in Southern New York. Annual, 1966-.

—— New York City and Its Hospitals:A Study of the Roles of the Municipal and Voluntary Hospitals Serving New York City. 1960.

—— Organized Ambulatory Medical Care Services. 1965.

—— A Study of Hospital Use, 1950 to 1962. 1964.

—— Study of Nurse Education Needs in the Southern New York Region. 1967.

—— A Study of Population Trends in New York City, Long Island and the Northern Metropolitan Region. 1963.

Health and Hospital Planning Council of Southern New York, Inc., and United Hospital Fund. A Partnership in Progress: The Affiliation Programs of the Municipal and Voluntary Hospitals Serving New York City. 1967.

Health Insurance Institute. Modern Health Insurance. New York, 1969.

—— Source Book of Health Insurance Data. New York, 1968.

Health Services Office, Community Action Program, Office of Economic Opportunity. The Comprehensive Neighborhood Health Services Program: Guidelines for Projects Submitted for Assistance under Section 222 (a) (4) (A) of the Economic Opportunity Act. Washington, D.C.: Office of Economic Opportunity, March, 1968.

Klarman, Herbert. Background, Issues and Policies in Health Services for the Aged in New York City. Report to the Interdepartmental Health Council of New York City, December, 1961.

—— Hospital Care in New York City. New York: Columbia University Press, 1963.

Lerner, Raymond, Corinne Kirchner, and Emil Dieckmann. New York City

Municipal General Hospital Outpatient Population Study, 1965. Reports Nos. 1-3. New York: School of Public Health and Administrative Medicine of Columbia University, various dates.

Levitan, Sar. "Healing the Poor: The Neighborhood Health Center." Washington, D.C.: Center for Manpower Policy Studies, August, 1968.

McLaughlin, Mary C. "Issues and Problems Associated with the Initiation of the Large Scale Ambulatory Care Program in New York City." Paper presented at the 95th Annual Meeting of the American Public Health Association, Miami Beach, Florida, October 23, 1967.

Mayor's Task Force on Medical Economics. *Report.* Paramus, N.J.: System Development Corporation, February 14, 1966.

Mayor's Task Force on Urban Design. *Threatened City: A Report on the Design of the City of New York.* (Paley Report). 1967.

Milbank Memorial Fund Quarterly. Vol. XLVI, No. 3 (July, 1968), Part I.

Muller, Charlotte, and Paul Worthington. "Factors Entering into Capital Decisions of Hospitals." Paper prepared for the Second Conference on the Economics of Health, December 5-7, 1968, at the Johns Hopkins University.

—— "The Time Structure of Capital Formation: Design and Construction of Municipal Hospital Projects," New York: Center for Social Research, City University of New York, 1968.

Parks, Robert, and Harvey Adelman. *System Analysis and Planning for Public Health Care in the City of New York.* Paramus, N.J.: System Development Corporation, March, 1966.

Piore, Nora. "Metropolitan Medical Economics," *Scientific American,* January, 1965.

Reed, J., and G. Reader. "Quantitative Survey of New York Hospital Emergency Room, 1965," *New York State Journal of Medicine,* May 15, 1967.

Rorem, C. Rufus. *Capital Financing for Hospitals.* New York: Health and Hospital Planning Council of Southern New York, 1968.

Rothstein, Peter. "The Closing of St. Francis Hospital: A Case Study of the Politics of Health Planning." New York: Health Policy Advisory Center, 1968.

Sayre, Wallace, and Herbert Kaufman. *Governing New York City: Politics in the Metropolis.* New York: W. W. Norton & Company, 1965.

School of Public Health and Administrative Medicine of Columbia University. *Charitable Institutions Budget, Hospital Medical Care, New York City, 1961-1964.* New York: School of Public Health and Administrative Medicine, May, 1965.

—— *Prepayment for Hospital Care in New York State: A Report on the Eight Blue Cross Plans Serving New York Residents.* New York: School of Public Health and Administrative Medicine, April, 1960.

—— *Prepayment for Medical and Dental Care in New York State: A Re-*

port on the Seven Blue Shield Plans, the Health Insurance Plan of Greater New York, Group Health Insurance, Inc., and Group Dental Insurance, Inc. Serving New York Residents. New York: School of Public Health and Administrative Medicine, October, 1962.

Somers, Anne, and Herman Somers. Medicare and the Hospitals. Washington, D.C.: Brookings Institution, 1967.

State of New York Commission of Investigation. Recommendations of the New York State Commission of Investigations Concerning New York City's Municipal Hospitals and the Affiliation Program. New York: State of New York Commission of Investigation, June, 1968.

Task Force on Health Manpower, National Commission on Community Health Services. Health Manpower. Washington, D.C.: Public Affairs Press, 1967.

Task Force on Tuberculosis Control in the United States. The Future of Tuberculosis Control: A Report to the Surgeon General of the Public Health Service by a Task Force on Tuberculosis Control in the United States. December, 1963.

Task Force on Tuberculosis in New York City. A Modern Attack on an Urban Health Problem. December, 1968.

Taylor, Vincent, and Joseph Newhouse. Improving Budgeting Procedures and Outpatient Operations in Nonprofit Hospitals. Santa Monica: Rand Corporation, 1970.

Technomics, Inc. Health Services in New York City: Problems, Policies and Programs. River Edge, N.J.: Technomics, Inc., August 7, 1967.

Teng, Clarence. The New York City Health Budget in Program Terms. Santa Monica: Rand Corporation, 1969.

Torrens, Paul. "The Impact of Emergency Services upon Patterns of Ambulatory Care." Report submitted to Medical Care Administrative Branch of Division of Community Health Services, Public Health Service, August, 1965.

Urban Medical Economics Research Project. Research Notes (a series of papers issued between 1962 and 1969 by various authors under the direction of Nora Piore).

—— A Profile of Physicians in the City of New York before Medicare and Medicaid. By Nora Piore and Sandra Sokol. New York: Urban Research Center of Hunter College, 1968.

INDEX